MW01533893

KIDNEY TRANSPLAN ı
AIR FRYER DIET
COOKBOOK

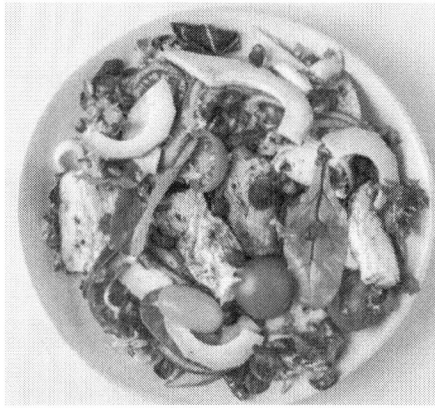

*Discover The Complete Nutritious And
Healthy Guide For Individuals In Managing
Renal Functions And Total Well-being*

Kathleen Scribner

DISCLAIMER

The recipes in this cookbook are designed solely for informative reasons. While every attempt has been taken to guarantee the correctness of the material, the author and publisher make no claims or warranties on the content's accuracy or completeness.

Readers should exercise caution and speak with a trained healthcare practitioner or nutritionist before making any dietary changes or attempting any of the recipes in this cookbook, particularly if they have certain dietary limitations, allergies, or medical concerns.

The author and publisher will not be held accountable for any loss, injury, or damage purportedly caused by any information or advice contained in this cookbook. Cooking and nutritional choices are personal, and readers are encouraged to make selections that reflect their own requirements and interests.

Enjoy exploring the recipes in this cookbook, but remember that your health and well-being come first.

TABLE OF CONTENTS

INTRODUCTION

Hello and welcome to the Kidney Transplant Air Fryer Diet Cookbook! I'm excited to share with you a compilation of tasty, healthy, and kidney-friendly dishes created exclusively for folks who have had a kidney transplant. This cookbook is about more than simply delivering safe and healthy meals for your condition; it is also about restoring joy and happiness to your dining table.

After a kidney transplant, it is critical to eat a diet that promotes health and recovery. This cookbook's recipes emphasize the use of nutritious grains, legumes, fresh fruits, and vegetables, all of which are high in fiber and essential for post-transplant health. Each meal is meticulously designed to be minimal in salt, potassium, and phosphorus, ensuring that you obtain the nutrients you require without taxing your new kidney.

Why an air fryer? Air frying is an excellent cooking method that allows you to enjoy crispy, tasty dishes without using excessive amounts of oil. It's a healthier alternative to standard frying and works well for making a range of foods fast and effortlessly. This cookbook includes a broad variety of tasty and kidney-friendly recipes, from breakfasts and snacks to main courses and desserts.

- This cookbook includes easy-to-follow cooking directions and nutritional information to help you make educated decisions.
- A wide selection of foods, including breakfasts, lunches, dinners, snacks, major meals, snacks and desserts.
- Tips for properly and safely utilizing your air fryer, among other things.

I hope these dishes encourage you to adopt a healthy, balanced diet that promotes kidney health while also satisfying your taste senses. Enjoy your culinary adventure with the Kidney Transplant Air Fryer Diet Cookbook, and here's to your health and happiness!

CHAPTER ONE: OVERVIEW OF THE KIDNEY TRANSPLANT DIET

Understanding the Kidney Transplant Diet

A kidney transplant is a life-changing treatment that allows many people with chronic kidney disease or end-stage renal disease to live a new life. However, it also entails the obligation of following a diet that promotes the health of the freshly transplanted kidney. The kidney transplant diet is intended to help your body recover and operate normally while also reducing complications including rejection, infection, and other health problems. Here's a thorough look at the major components and concepts of the kidney transplant diet:

1. Hydration

Staying hydrated is essential for kidney health. Proper hydration allows the kidneys to filter waste and maintain electrolyte balance. However, excessive hydration might stress the kidneys. Your healthcare professional will offer you fluid intake suggestions that are tailored to your personal needs.

2. Protein

Following a kidney transplant, your body requires enough protein to mend and rebuild tissues. However, consuming too much protein can put a burden on the kidneys. It is essential to ingest the recommended quantity of protein, which may be assessed by your healthcare professional. Poultry, fish, and eggs are good sources of lean protein, as are plant-based proteins such as beans and lentils.

3. Sodium

Sodium can promote fluid retention and raise blood pressure, which can be bad for your kidneys. Limiting salt consumption promotes healthy blood pressure and fluid balance. Choose fresh meals over processed ones, season with herbs and spices rather than salt, and read product labels to keep track of sodium levels.

4. Potassium

Potassium is a vital element, but following a kidney donation, its levels must be carefully monitored. Both high and low potassium levels can be harmful. Apples, berries, green beans, and carrots are examples of fruits and vegetables with intermediate potassium levels, but high-potassium foods such as bananas, oranges, and potatoes should be avoided.

5. Phosphorus

High phosphorus levels can cause bone and cardiovascular concerns. Post-transplant patients frequently need to decrease their phosphorus intake. This can be accomplished by eliminating high-phosphorus foods such as dairy products, nuts, seeds, and carbonated beverages. Instead, choose low-phosphorus options and see your nutritionist for precise advice.

6. Healthy Fats

Healthy fats are beneficial to general health but should be used in moderation. Concentrate on the unsaturated fats found in olive oil, avocados, almonds, and fatty seafood. These fats promote heart health without putting an additional load on the kidneys.

7. Carbohydrates

Managing blood sugar levels is critical, especially if you are using immunosuppressive drugs that might impair glucose metabolism. Choose complex carbs with a low glycemic index, such as whole grains, veggies, and legumes. These give long-lasting energy and assist in keeping blood sugar levels constant.

8. Fiber

A high-fiber diet promotes digestive health and regulates blood sugar levels. Include whole grains, legumes, fruits, and vegetables in your diet to guarantee optimal fiber consumption. Fiber also improves satiety, which helps you manage your weight.

9. Vitamins And Minerals

Certain drugs may impact vitamin and mineral absorption following a kidney transplant. A well-balanced, nutrient-dense diet is crucial. However, unless prescribed by your healthcare professional, avoid using over-the-counter vitamins, as some may conflict with your prescriptions.

10. Preventing Foodborne Illness

Immunosuppressive drugs might increase your susceptibility to infections. Practice food safety by properly washing fruits and vegetables, cooking meats to acceptable temperatures, avoiding raw or undercooked meals, and keeping your kitchen clean.

11. Alcohol & Caffeine

Both alcohol and caffeine should be used in moderation. Excessive alcohol consumption can impair liver function and interfere with medicine, but too much caffeine can induce dehydration and influence blood pressure. Consult your healthcare practitioner to establish appropriate dosages for your case.

12. Tracking and Adjusting Your Diet

Regular check-ups with your doctor and nutritionist are necessary for monitoring your kidney function and nutritional condition. They will provide you with tailored guidance and change your diet as needed to ensure it matches your changing health requirements.

Understanding and following the kidney transplant diet is critical to the long-term success of your transplant. Making educated dietary choices and following the advice offered by your healthcare team can help you maintain kidney health, improve your quality of
life, and reap the advantages of your new kidney.

Benefits of Kidney Transplant Diet Using an Air Fryer

The kidney transplant diet is critical for the longevity and health of the transplanted kidney. Incorporating an air fryer into this diet may provide various advantages, making the diet not only healthier but also more pleasurable and sustainable. Here's a thorough look at the main advantages of utilizing an air fryer.

1. Reduced Fat Consumption

One of the key advantages of utilizing an air fryer is that it significantly reduces fat consumption.

Traditional frying methods use a lot of oil, which can be harmful to your kidneys. Air fryers utilize little to no oil, which reduces calorie and fat consumption while maintaining the ideal crispiness and flavor.

2. Improved Nutrient Retention

Air frying preserves nutrients in meals better than other cooking methods. Traditional techniques, which use high heat and extensive cooking times, might destroy vitamins and minerals. Air frying cooks food rapidly and retains its nutritious nutrients.

3. Improved Heart Health

A diet low in harmful fats and high in nutrients promotes heart health, which is especially important for kidney transplant patients. Air-fried meals are lower in trans fats and cholesterol, which benefits cardiovascular health.

4. Convenience and Ease of Use

Air fryers are user-friendly and need little preparation and cleaning, making it simpler for people to keep to their diets. This ease promotes regular, healthy eating habits.

5. Flexibility in Cooking

Air fryers can cook a variety of meals, including vegetables, meats, and sweets. This adaptability contributes to a diverse and fascinating diet, minimizing dietary tiredness.

6. Improved Blood Sugar Control

Managing blood sugar levels is critical for kidney transplant patients, especially if they are on immunosuppressive medicines that influence glucose metabolism. Air frying lowers the glycemic load of meals compared to conventional frying.

Fiona's Transformation with the Air Fryer

Fiona, a 45-year-old kidney transplant recipient, struggled to adjust her diet following surgery. The conventional frying methods she preferred were no longer available, and she found it difficult to enjoy her meals. Fiona, determined to better her health, purchased an air fryer. She was first hesitant, but quickly became a fan. She began with easy recipes like air-fried zucchini chips and then progressed to more difficult ones like quinoa breakfast bowls and stuffed bell peppers.

The Benefits:

1. Reduced Fat Intake: Fiona's air-fried foods were much lower in fat, allowing her to maintain a healthy weight without placing further strain on her kidneys.

2. Nutrient Preservation: Air-fried veggies retained more nutrients, which enhanced her total nutrition.

3. Heart Health: By eliminating harmful fats, Fiona improved her cardiovascular health, which was critical for her post-transplant recovery.

4. Convenience: Fiona was able to keep to her diet thanks to the air fryer's simplicity of use and quick cleaning.

5. Variety: The air fryer's adaptability ensured that her meals were varied and enjoyable.

6. Blood Sugar Control: Fiona found that air frying helped her regulate her blood sugar levels more effectively, which reduced the effects of her immunosuppressive drugs.

Fiona's health improved dramatically. She felt more energized, her test results improved, and she was able to enjoy her meals without the shame or health dangers that come with regular frying. The air fryer had altered her diet, and thereby her life.

Using an air fryer as part of a kidney transplant diet has several advantages, including lowering harmful fats, retaining nutrients, and boosting overall ease and adaptability in the kitchen. Fiona's experience demonstrates how a simple kitchen gadget might help her maintain a b better, more pleasant diet after transplant.

Food To Embrace and Avoid

After a kidney transplant, your diet is critical to preserving the health of your new kidney, supporting your general well-being, and avoiding problems. Understanding which foods to eat and which to avoid will help you make informed dietary decisions that promote lifespan and excellent kidney function after transplantation. Here is a full overview of the foods you should embrace and avoid:

Foods To Embrace

1. Lean Proteins

- Examples include chicken, turkey, fish, eggs, tofu, and beans.
- **Benefits:** Lean proteins, which are necessary for tissue repair and immunological function, are gentler on the kidneys than high-fat proteins. They supply the required amino acids while avoiding excessive fat.

2. Whole Grains

- Examples include brown rice, quinoa, barley, oatmeal, and whole wheat bread.
- **Benefits:** Whole grains are abundant in fiber, which helps manage blood sugar levels and improves digestive health. They also supply critical vitamins and minerals.

3. Fruits And Vegetables

- Examples include apples, berries, pears, green beans, carrots, and spinach (in moderation).

- **Benefits:** Fruits and vegetables are high in vitamins, minerals, and antioxidants, which promote general health and kidney function. They contribute to a balanced diet and supply essential nutrients.

4. Healthy Fats

- Examples include olive oil, avocado, almonds, and seeds.
- **Benefits:** Healthy fats promote heart health and minimize inflammation. They supply necessary fatty acids, which are important to general health.

5. Low-fat Dairy Or Dairy Alternatives

- Examples include low-fat milk, yogurt, and cheese, as well as plant-based equivalents such as almond milk and soy yogurt.
- **Benefits:** These foods provide calcium and vitamin D, which are essential for bone health. To limit your saturated fat intake, use low-fat or plant-based choices.

6. High-Fiber Foods

- Examples include lentils, chickpeas, broccoli, and whole grain items.

- Benefits: Fiber regulates blood sugar levels and promotes digestive health. High-fiber meals might also help you maintain a healthy weight.

7. Hydrating Fluids

- Examples include water, herbal teas, and infused water (including cucumber, lemon, or mint).
- Benefits: Staying hydrated allows the kidney to operate properly and maintains electrolyte balance. Adequate fluid consumption is necessary for good health.

Foods To Avoid

1. High-sodium Foods

- Examples include processed meats (bacon, sausages), canned soups, fast meals, and salty snacks like chips and pretzels.
- Risks: Excess salt intake can cause fluid retention and high blood pressure, which can strain the

kidneys. Limiting salt intake helps to maintain good kidney function.

2. High Potassium Foods

- Examples include bananas, oranges, potatoes, tomatoes, and spinach.
- **Risks:** Excess potassium can result in hyperkalemia, which impairs heart rhythm and muscle function. Monitoring potassium intake is critical for kidney transplant patients.

3. High-Phosphorus Foods

- Examples include dairy products, almonds, seeds, and cola drinks.
- **Risks:** Elevated phosphorus levels can cause bone and cardiovascular disorders. Limiting phosphorus consumption promotes bone health and prevents hardening of blood vessels.

4. High-fat And Fried Foods

- Examples include fried chicken, French fries, doughnuts, and other deep-fried dishes.

- **Risks:** Consuming these foods can lead to weight gain, high cholesterol, and cardiovascular disease. Avoiding high-fat meals promotes a healthy weight and cardiovascular health.

5. Sugar-containing Foods And Beverages

- Examples include sodas, sweets, pastries, and sugary cereals.
- **Risks:** Consuming too much sugar can cause weight gain and blood sugar surges, which are especially dangerous for individuals using immunosuppressive drugs. Limiting sugar consumption helps control blood sugar levels and reduces weight gain.

6. Processed And Packaged Foods

- Examples include instant noodles, frozen foods, snacks and bars.
- **Risks:** These foods frequently include excessive amounts of salt, preservatives, and harmful fats. Reduced intake of processed foods benefits both general health and renal function.

7. Alcohol and Caffeine (in excess)

- Examples include alcoholic beverages, coffee, and energy drinks.
- **Risks:** Drinking too much alcohol or coffee might dehydrate you and interfere with your prescriptions. Moderation is essential for maintaining sufficient hydration and preventing unfavorable drug interactions.

Understanding and following the dietary guidelines for kidney transplant patients is critical to the long-term effectiveness of the transplant. You may have a better, more meaningful life after transplant by making educated eating choices and according to healthcare professionals' recommendations.

Recommend Nutrient Intake

Maintaining a healthy diet is critical for kidney transplant patients to guarantee the donated kidney's health and lifespan, as well as improve general well-being. Here are the main recommended nutritional intakes for kidney transplant patients:

1. Protein

- The recommended daily intake is 0.8 to 1.0 grams per kilogram of body weight.
- Protein sources include lean meats, chicken, fish, eggs, tofu, and lentils.
- **Importance:** An adequate protein intake is required for tissue repair and immunological function. However, too much protein can stress the kidneys, so balance is essential.

2. Sodium

- **Recommended Daily Intake**: less than 2,300 milligrams.
- **Ingredients**: Fresh produce, herbs, and spices. Avoid processed meals and salty goods.
- **Importance:** Limiting salt intake helps maintain blood pressure and reduces fluid retention, which can stress the kidneys.

3. Potassium

- **Recommended Daily Intake:** 2,000 to 3,000 milligrams, however this might vary depending on test findings.
- **Sources:** Moderate potassium foods include apples, berries, green beans, and carrots. Avoid potassium-rich foods such as bananas and potatoes.
- **Importance:** Maintaining adequate potassium levels is essential for heart function and muscle contraction. Both high and low potassium levels can be detrimental.

4. Phosphorus

- The recommended daily intake is 800 to 1,000 mg.
- Foods low in phosphorus include fresh fruits and vegetables, as well as grains. Avoid phosphorus-rich foods such as dairy products, nuts, and seeds.
- **Importance:** Maintaining phosphorus levels can help avoid bone disease and cardiovascular problems. High phosphorus levels can cause calcification in blood vessels and organs.

5. Calcium

- The recommended daily intake is 1,000 to 1,200 milligrams.
- Sources include low-fat dairy products and fortified plant-based equivalents such as almond milk and tofu.
- **Importance:** Calcium is necessary for bone health. Adequate intake helps to prevent osteoporosis, a concern associated with immunosuppressive medicines.

6. Fluids

- **Recommended Intake:** Varies according to individual needs, but often 2 to 3 liters daily.
- Sources include water, herbal teas, and low-potassium fruit juices.
- **Importance**: Staying hydrated is essential for kidney function. Proper hydration allows the kidneys to filter waste and maintain electrolyte balance.

7. Fiber

- The recommended daily intake is 25-30 grams.
- Sources include whole grains, fruits, vegetables, and legumes.

- **Importance:** Fiber boosts digestive health, regulates blood sugar levels, and increases satiety, all of which benefit weight management.

8. Vitamins And Minerals

- **Recommended Intake**: Based on individual requirements and medical guidance.
- **Sources:** A well-balanced diet that includes fruits, vegetables, and whole grains. Unless specifically recommended, avoid over-the-counter supplements.
- **Importance:** Some drugs might interfere with vitamin and mineral absorption. A balanced diet guarantees optimal nutritional intake while avoiding excessive supplementation, which can be hazardous.

9. Healthy Fats

- The recommended intake is 20-35% of total daily calories.
- Sources include olive oil, avocados, almonds, and seeds.
- **Importance**: Healthy fats promote heart health and reduce inflammation. They supply vital fatty acids, which promote general health.

10. Sugars

- The recommended intake is less than 10% of total daily calories.
- Natural sources include fruits and small amounts of honey or maple syrup. Avoid processed meals with extra sugars.
- **Importance:** Limiting sugar intake helps regulate blood sugar levels, which is especially essential for individuals using immunosuppressive drugs that might impair glucose metabolism.

By following these dietary recommendations, kidney transplant patients can help their new kidney's health, lower the chance of complications, and improve their overall quality of life. It is critical to collaborate closely with healthcare practitioners and nutritionists to adjust these suggestions to specific requirements and medical situations.

CHAPTER TWO: BEGINNING YOUR KIDNEY TRANSPLANT AIR FRYER JOURNEY

Essential Kitchen Tools and Equipment

Going on a kidney transplant air fryer path entails adopting dietary modifications that benefit your new kidney and general health. Equipping your kitchen with the necessary tools and equipment will make the move easier and more pleasurable. Here's a full list of the key kitchen gear and equipment you'll need:

1. Air Fryer

- Why It's Essential: The air fryer is the foundation of your new cooking method. It enables you to make tasty, crispy dishes with less oil, lowering fat consumption and improving heart health.
- Look for adjustable temperature settings, a timer, a nonstick basket, and a large enough capacity to make meals for your family.

2. Digital Food Scale

- Why It's Important: Accurately measuring portion sizes and components is critical for controlling your nutritional consumption, particularly protein, salt, and potassium.
- Features to Look for: Digital display, tare function, and measurement in grams and ounces.

3. Measuring Cup And Spoon

- **Why It's Important:** Precise ingredient measurements guarantee that you follow dietary requirements and maintain the proper nutritional balance.
- **Features to Look For:** Durable, simple to clean, and with clearly indicated measures.

4. Cutting Boards

- **Why It's Necessary**: A strong cutting board is required for securely preparing fruits, vegetables, and other foods.
- Look for a non-slip surface that is simple to clean, as well as separate boards for raw meats and vegetables to prevent cross-contamination.

5. Sharp Knives

- **Why It's Important:** Sharp knives allow you to prepare ingredients swiftly and safely, lowering the danger of mishaps.
- Look for a high-quality chef's knife, paring knife, and serrated knife for versatility.

6. Mixing Bowls

- **Why It's Important:** Mixing bowls are used to combine ingredients, marinate, and prepare batters.
- **Features to Look For:** A variety of sizes, preferably in stainless steel or glass for durability and ease of cleaning.

7. Silicone Spatulas And Tongs

- **Why It's Important:** Silicone tools are heat-resistant and won't harm your air fryer's non-stick surface.
- Look for features like durability, heat resistance, and ease of cleaning.

8. Non-stick Spray or Oil Mist

- **Why It's Important:** Using only a small amount of oil minimizes sticking and promotes uniform cooking in the air fryer.
- **Features to Look For:** A high-quality, refillable oil mister or nonstick cooking spray that allows you to adjust the quantity of oil used.

9. Vegetable Peeler

- **Why It's Important:** A vegetable peeler is important for prepping fruits and vegetables so they're ready to cook or consume raw.
- **Features to Look for:** An ergonomic grip and a sharp blade for effective peeling.

10. Parchment Paper

- **Why It's Important:** Using parchment paper to line the air fryer basket simplifies cleanup and prevents sticking.
- **Features to Look For**: Pre-cut sheets or a roll that may be trimmed to size, assuring air fryer safety and heat resistance.

11. Oven-safe Baking Dishes And Ramekins

- **Why It's Important:** These are required for producing baked foods, individual portions, and desserts in the air fryer.
- **Features to Look For:** Dishes and ramekins that fit easily within your air fryer basket and are made of high-temperature resistant materials.

12. Food Processor Or Blender

- **Why it's essential:** For quick and efficient purees, batters, and vegetable chopping.
- Look for features like several speed settings, sturdy blades, and a big capacity.

13. Thermometer

- **Why It's Important:** Making sure meat and other items are cooked to the appropriate temperature is critical for food safety.
- **Features to Look For:** Instant-read digital thermometer provides rapid and precise readings.

14. Storage Containers

- **Why It's Important:** Proper storage of prepared items and leftovers preserves freshness and makes meal preparation faster.
- **Features to Look For:** Airtight, BPA-free containers come in a variety of sizes for maximum usability.

Additional Tips for Kitchen Setup

1. Organize Your Kitchen: Make sure your tools and equipment are conveniently accessible. An organized kitchen helps to expedite the cooking process and improves meal preparation efficiency.

2. Plan Your Meal: Use your equipment to prepare items ahead of time. Planning meals ahead of time allows you to stick to your dietary limits while also reducing the burden of everyday meal preparation.

3. Label and Date Food: Use labels to record the date the food was produced or opened. This approach promotes food freshness and decreases waste.

4. Keep a Recipe Book or App: Having a library of kidney-friendly dishes on hand may provide inspiration and make meal planning and preparation easier. There are various applications and publications designed expressly for kidney-friendly diets.

By stocking your kitchen with these necessary tools and equipment, you may properly manage your kidney transplant diet while also enjoying tasty, healthy meals. An air fryer, when paired with the appropriate accessories, will make your cooking experience easier, healthier, and more fun.

Air Fryer Basics and Safety Tips

Starting your kidney transplant air fryer adventure entails not only learning the nutritional needs but also knowing how to operate your air fryer safely and efficiently. Here's a complete tutorial on the fundamentals of operating an air fryer, as well as important safety guidelines to get you started:

1. How an Air Fryer Works

An air fryer is a kitchen equipment that cooks food by blowing hot air through it. This method cooks the food using convection, which results in a crispy coating comparable to frying but with substantially less oil. The fast air circulation cooks food evenly and rapidly, giving it a healthier option than traditional frying techniques.

2. Setting Up Your Air Fryer

- **Placement:** Place the air fryer on a level, heat-resistant surface with enough room for airflow. Make sure it isn't near any combustible stuff.
- **Initial Cleaning:** Before using the air fryer, clean the basket and any detachable parts with warm soapy water and thoroughly dry.
- **Assembly:** Reassemble the air fryer using the manufacturer's instructions.

3. Basic Operation

- **Preheating:** Heat the air fryer for 3-5 minutes before adding food to guarantee consistent frying.
- **Temperature Settings**: Most air fryers include temperature controls that range from 180°F to 400°F (82°C to 204°C). Adjust the temperature to meet the recipe's specifications.
- **Cooking Time**: Cooking times differ according to the kind and quantity of food. For precise timing, see the air fryer instructions and recipe recommendations.
- **Shaking or Turning Food**: To ensure equal cooking, shake the basket or turn the food halfway through the cooking period.

Safety Tips

1. **Read The Manual**

- **Importance:** Each air fryer model is unique. Reading the user manual can help you grasp the exact features, settings, and safety measures of your device.

2. **Avoid Overcrowding**

- **Why:** Overcrowding the basket might cause uneven cooking. Allow adequate space for air to flow around each item of food.
-**Tips:** Cook in batches as necessary to ensure meal quality.

3. **Use Heat-resistant Tools**

- **Why:** During frying, the air fryer's basket and inside get extremely hot. Use heat-resistant gloves and utensils to handle the basket and food.
- **Tip:** Silicone or wooden utensils are good since they will not ruin the nonstick coating.

4. Regular Cleaning

- **Why:** Regular cleaning minimizes the accumulation of oil and food particles, which can impair performance and safety.
- **How:** After each usage, thoroughly clean the basket, tray, and other detachable pieces with warm soapy water. Wipe the outside and inside with a wet cloth.

5. Track Cooking Progress

- **Why:** Although air fryers are intended to be safe, it is critical to watch the cooking process to avoid overcooking or burning.
- **Tip:** Check the meal regularly and adjust the time and temperature accordingly.

6. Use On A Stable Surface

- **Why:** Placing the air fryer on a sturdy, level surface reduces tipping and mishaps.
- **Tips:** Avoid putting the air fryer near the edge of the counter.

7. Allow Cooling Time

- **Why:** The air fryer and its components stay hot after cooking. Allow it to cool before handling or cleaning.
- **Tip:** After usage, unplug the air fryer and allow it to cool fully before storing it.

8. Proper Ventilation

- **Why:** Air fryers require adequate ventilation to perform properly and safely. Make sure there is enough room around the device so that air can flow.
- **Tip:** Do not use the air fryer in restricted places or near walls.

9. Avoid Aerosol Cooking Sprays

- **Why:** Aerosol cooking sprays can ruin the basket's nonstick coating.
- **Tip:** Apply oil to the food using a pump spray bottle or by brushing it on lightly.

10. Check for Damage

- **Why:** Regularly examine the power wire and plug for damage. Using a faulty air fryer might result in electrical dangers.
- **Tip:** If you notice any damage, stop using the product and contact the manufacturer or a skilled technician for repairs.

Getting the Most Out of Your Air Fryer

1. Experiment With Recipes

- **Why:** The air fryer's adaptability allows you to cook a variety of foods. Experimenting allows you to find new recipes that meet your kidney-friendly diet.
- **Tip:** Begin with easy recipes and progress to more complicated meals as you get more familiar with the device.

2. Adjust Cooking Times and Temperatures

- **Why:** Air fryers cook food more quickly than traditional techniques. To avoid overcooking, adjust the cooking time and temperature.
- **Tip:** For air fryer model-specific recommendations, consult recipe books or internet resources.

3. Use Parchment Paper or Silicone Liners

- **Why:** These liners reduce stickiness and make cleanup easier.
- **Tip:** Make sure the liners have perforations for adequate air circulation.

4. Preheat for Optimal Results

- **Why**: Preheating promotes uniform cooking and improves texture.
- **Tip:** Preheat the air fryer to the proper temperature and let it run for 3-5 minutes before adding the food.

5. Shake or Turn Food to Ensure Even Cooking

- **Why:** Shaking or turning the food guarantees that it is cooked evenly on all sides.
- **Tip:** Use a timer to remind yourself to shake or turn the meal halfway through the cooking process.

You may begin your kidney transplant air fryer adventure with confidence if you grasp the fundamentals of air fryer operation and follow these safety guidelines. This technique will assist you in preparing nutritious, delicious meals while guaranteeing your safety and utilizing the benefits of your gadget.

CHAPTER THREE: QUICK AND EASY KIDNEY TRANSPLANT AIR FRYER BREAKFAST RECIPES

Good morning, and welcome to your nutritious and tasty breakfast recipes. Begin your day with meals that are not only delicious but also designed to promote renal health. Each breakfast meal is simple to create with your air fryer, delivering the ideal balance of nutrition and flavor. Dive into these delectable breakfast alternatives to energize your mornings the best way!

1. Air Fryer Oatmeal Cups

Ingredients:

- 1 cup rolled oats
- 1/2 cup unsweetened applesauce
- 1/4 cup honey or maple syrup
- 1/4 cup almond milk (or any low-potassium milk alternative)
- 1 tsp vanilla extract
- 1 tsp ground cinnamon
- 1/4 tsp salt
- 1/2 cup mixed berries (blueberries, raspberries, strawberries)
- 1/4 cup chopped nuts (walnuts or almonds)

Instructions:

1. Place the rolled oats, almond milk, honey (or maple syrup), unsweetened applesauce, ground cinnamon, vanilla extract, and salt in a large mixing dish. Stir thoroughly to include all of the ingredients.

2. Ensure that the chopped nuts and mixed berries are uniformly distributed throughout the oatmeal mixture by folding them in.

3. Use non-stick spray to lightly oil a muffin pan or silicone muffin cups.

4. Fill approximately 3/4 of the muffin cups with the oatmeal mixture using a spoon. To make sure the mixture is compact, gently press down.

5. Set the air fryer's temperature for three minutes at 350°F/175°C.

6. To ensure enough air circulation, place the muffin cups in the air fryer basket, making sure they do not touch.

7. Air fry the oatmeal cups for 12 to 15 minutes, or until they are firm to the touch and have a golden brown top, at 350°F (175°C).

8. Take out of the air fryer and allow the oatmeal cups to rest in the muffin cups for a few minutes before moving them to a wire rack to cool entirely.

9. Savor warm or at room temperature the oatmeal cups. Any leftovers can be kept in the fridge for up to five days if they are kept in an airtight container.

Nutritional Information (per oatmeal cup, based on 10 servings):

- **Calories: 110**
- **Protein: 2g**
- **Carbohydrates: 20g**
- **Dietary Fiber: 3g**
- **Sugars: 8g**
- **Total Fat: 3g**
- **Saturated Fat: 0.5g**
- **Sodium: 60mg**
- **Potassium: 100mg**

2. Veggie-Packed Breakfast Frittata

Ingredients:

- 6 large eggs
- 1/4 cup almond milk (or any low-potassium milk alternative)
- 1/2 cup chopped spinach
- 1/2 cup diced bell peppers (any color)
- 1/4 cup diced onions
- 1/2 cup cherry tomatoes, halved
- 1/4 cup shredded low-fat cheese (optional)
- 1/2 tsp garlic powder
- 1/2 tsp onion powder
- 1/4 tsp black pepper
- 1/4 tsp salt
- Non-stick spray

Instructions:

1. Beat the eggs and almond milk together thoroughly in a large mixing dish.
2. To the egg mixture, add the chopped spinach, diced onions, bell peppers, and cherry tomatoes. If using, add the shredded cheese. Stir until every veggie is dispersed equally.

3. Add the salt, black pepper, onion powder, and garlic powder to the mixture and whisk to blend in the ingredients.

4. Use non-stick spray to lightly coat a circular cake pan or oven-safe dish that fits within the air fryer basket.

5. Evenly distribute the egg and veggie mixture into the prepared dish.

6. Set the air fryer's temperature for three minutes at 350°F/175°C.

7. Put the dish in the air fryer basket and cook for 15 to 20 minutes at 350°F (175°C), or until the frittata is set in the middle and has a light brown crust. If you stick a toothpick into the middle to check for doneness, it should come out clean.

8. Before slicing and serving, carefully take the dish out of the air fryer and allow the frittata to cool for a few minutes.

9. Eat the frittata warm, and keep any leftovers in the fridge for up to three days in an airtight container.

Nutritional Information (per serving, based on 6 servings):

- **Calories: 120**
- **Protein: 9g**
- **Carbohydrates: 4g**
- **Dietary Fiber: 1g**

- **Sugars: 2g**
- **Total Fat: 8g**
- **Saturated Fat: 2g**
- **Sodium: 180mg**
- **Potassium: 250mg**

3. Air Fryer Sweet Potato Hash

Ingredients:

- 2 medium sweet potatoes, peeled and diced into small cubes
- 1/2 red bell pepper, diced
- 1/2 green bell pepper, diced
- 1 small onion, diced
- 1 tbsp olive oil
- 1/2 tsp garlic powder
- 1/2 tsp paprika
- 1/4 tsp black pepper
- 1/4 tsp salt
- Fresh parsley for garnish (optional)

Instructions:

1. For three minutes, preheat the air fryer to 375°F (190°C).
2. Add the onion, bell peppers, and cubed sweet potatoes to a large mixing basin.

3. Pour the olive oil over the veggies and toss to ensure that they are uniformly coated.

4. Top the mixture with a sprinkle of salt, black pepper, paprika, and garlic powder. To make sure the seasonings are dispersed equally, toss one more.

5. Use a tiny bit of olive oil or non-stick spray to gently oil the air fryer basket.

6. Evenly distribute the spiced vegetable mixture into the air fryer basket.

7. To achieve consistent cooking, air fry for 15 to 20 minutes at 375°F (190°C), shaking the basket halfway through.

8. Use a fork to pierce a sweet potato cube to check for doneness; it should be soft and have a hint of crunch on the exterior.

9. Transfer the sweet potato hash to a serving plate after carefully taking it out of the air fryer.

10. If wanted, garnish with fresh parsley and serve warm.

Nutritional Information (per serving, based on 4 servings):

- **Calories: 130**
- **Protein: 2g**
- **Carbohydrates: 26g**
- **Dietary Fiber: 4g**
- **Sugars: 7g**
- **Total Fat: 4g**

- **Saturated Fat: 0.5g**
- **Sodium: 150mg**
- **Potassium: 450mg**

4. Air Fryer Fruit and Nut Granola

Ingredients:

- 2 cups rolled oats
- 1/2 cup chopped nuts (almonds, walnuts, or pecans)
- 1/2 cup dried fruit (raisins, cranberries, or apricots)
- 1/4 cup unsweetened coconut flakes (optional)
- 1/4 cup honey or maple syrup
- 1/4 cup coconut oil or olive oil
- 1 tsp vanilla extract
- 1 tsp ground cinnamon
- 1/4 tsp salt

Instructions:

1. For three minutes, preheat the air fryer to 300°F (150°C).
2. Place the chopped nuts, dried fruit, rolled oats, and unsweetened coconut flakes (if using) in a large mixing dish.

3. Melt the honey (or maple syrup) and coconut oil (or olive oil) in a small saucepan over low heat. Add the salt, ground cinnamon, and vanilla essence and stir until thoroughly blended.

4. After thoroughly mixing to make sure everything is coated equally, pour the liquid mixture over the oat mixture.

5. To stop the granola from dropping through the openings, line the air fryer basket with parchment paper.

6. Evenly distribute the granola blend into the lined air fryer basket.

7. To achieve consistent cooking, air fry for 10 to 15 minutes at 300°F (150°C), shaking the basket every five minutes. To avoid burning it, pay great attention to it.

8. Carefully take the granola out of the air fryer and place it on a large baking sheet to cool entirely once it is crispy and golden brown. As it cools, it will get crisper still.

9. You may keep the cooled granola for up to two weeks at room temperature in an airtight jar.

Nutritional Information (per serving, based on 8 servings):

- **Calories: 200**
- **Protein: 4g**
- **Carbohydrates: 28g**

- **Dietary Fiber: 4g**
- **Sugars: 10g**
- **Total Fat: 9g**
- **Saturated Fat: 4g**
- **Sodium: 60mg**
- **Potassium: 150mg**

5. Avocado and Tomato Toast

Ingredients:

- 2 slices whole-grain bread
- 1 ripe avocado
- 1 medium tomato, sliced
- 1/4 tsp garlic powder
- 1/4 tsp black pepper
- 1/8 tsp salt
- 1/2 tsp lemon juice
- Fresh basil leaves for garnish (optional)

Instructions:

1. For three minutes, preheat the air fryer to 350°F (175°C).
2. In the air fryer, toast the whole-grain bread pieces gently for three to five minutes, or until they are as crispy as you like.

3. Slice the avocado in half, take out the pit, and scoop out the flesh into a bowl while the bread is toasting.

4. Using a fork, mash the avocado until it has a creamy texture. Incorporate the lemon juice, salt, black pepper, and garlic powder, blending well.

5. After the bread is toasted, take it out of the air fryer and cover each piece evenly with mashed avocado.

6. Evenly distribute the tomato slices on the bread and place them on top of the avocado.

7. You may optionally add fresh basil leaves as a garnish to give the dish more taste and color.

8. Present right away and savor.

Nutritional Information (per serving, based on 2 servings):

- **Calories: 250**
- **Protein: 6g**
- **Carbohydrates: 30g**
- **Dietary Fiber: 10g**
- **Sugars: 4g**
- **Total Fat: 15g**
- **Saturated Fat: 2g**
- **Sodium: 230mg**
- **Potassium: 700mg**

6. Air Fryer Banana Oat Pancakes

Ingredients:

- 1 cup rolled oats
- 1 ripe banana
- 1/2 cup almond milk (or any low-potassium milk alternative)
- 1 large egg
- 1 tsp baking powder
- 1/2 tsp vanilla extract
- 1/4 tsp ground cinnamon
- 1/8 tsp salt
- Non-stick spray

Instructions:

1. Process the rolled oats in a food processor or blender until they resemble fine flour.
2. Fill the blender with the ripe banana, egg, almond milk, baking powder, vanilla essence, powdered cinnamon, and salt. Blend the ingredients until it's fully incorporated and smooth.
3. Set the air fryer's temperature for three minutes to 350°F/175°C.
4. Lightly use non-stick spray to coat a silicone muffin cup or small round baking dish that fits into your air fryer.

5. Transfer around 1/4 cup of the mixture into the baking dish or muffin cup, leveling it out to create a pancake.

6. Insert the baking dish or muffin cup filled with food into the air fryer basket.

7. Air fry the pancake for 8 to 10 minutes, or until it sets and the top turns golden brown, at 350°F/175°C.

8. Take the pancake out of the air fryer with care, then place it on a platter. Proceed to steps 5-7 using the leftover batter.

9. You can choose to serve the pancakes warm with fresh fruit, nuts or seeds, and a drizzle of honey or maple syrup on top.

Nutritional Information (per serving, based on 4 servings):

- **Calories: 120**
- **Protein: 4g**
- **Carbohydrates: 20g**
- **Dietary Fiber: 3g**
- **Sugars: 5g**
- **Total Fat: 3g**
- **Saturated Fat: 0.5g**
- **Sodium: 150mg**
- **Potassium: 200mg**

7. Spinach and Mushroom Breakfast Wrap

Ingredients:

- 1 whole-grain tortilla
- 1 cup fresh spinach leaves
- 1/2 cup sliced mushrooms
- 2 large eggs
- 1/4 cup shredded low-fat cheese (optional)
- 1/4 tsp garlic powder
- 1/4 tsp black pepper
- 1/8 tsp salt
- 1 tbsp olive oil
- Non-stick spray

Instructions:

1. For three minutes, preheat the air fryer to 350°F (175°C).
2. Heat the olive oil in a medium-sized pan over medium heat.
3. Add the sliced mushrooms to the skillet and cook for 3–4 minutes, or until they begin to soften.
4. Cook the fresh spinach leaves in the pan for one to two minutes, or until they have wilted.

5. In a small bowl, thoroughly mix the eggs with the salt, black pepper, and garlic powder.

6. Push the mushrooms and spinach to one side of the skillet, then transfer the eggs into the vacant space, scrambling them until they are well cooked.

7. Combine the cooked eggs with the mushrooms and spinach.

8. Lay the whole-grain tortilla out flat, and if you're using it, scatter the shredded cheese in the middle.

9. Evenly distribute the spinach, mushroom, and egg mixture onto the tortilla with a spoon.

10. Tightly roll the tortilla into a wrap, tucking in the edges to hold the filling in place.

11. Insert the wrap into the air fryer basket after giving it a quick spritz of non-stick spray.

12. Air fry the tortilla for five to seven minutes, or until it is crispy and golden brown, at 350°F/175°C.

13. Take the breakfast wrap out of the air fryer with care, allow it to cool for a minute, and then cut it in two.

14. Warm up and savor.

Nutritional Information (per serving, based on 1 wrap):

- **Calories: 300**
- **Protein: 17g**
- **Carbohydrates: 30g**
- **Dietary Fiber: 6g**

- Sugars: 2g
- Total Fat: 12g
- Saturated Fat: 3g
- Sodium: 450mg
- Potassium: 500mg

8. Air Fryer Apple Cinnamon Muffins

Ingredients:

- 1 cup whole wheat flour
- 1/2 cup rolled oats
- 1/2 cup unsweetened applesauce
- 1/4 cup honey or maple syrup
- 1/4 cup almond milk (or any low-potassium milk alternative)
- 1 large egg
- 1 medium apple, peeled and finely chopped
- 1 tsp baking powder
- 1/2 tsp baking soda
- 1 tsp ground cinnamon
- 1/4 tsp salt
- 1/4 tsp vanilla extract
- Non-stick spray

Instructions:

1. For three minutes, preheat the air fryer to 350°F (175°C).

2. Place the whole wheat flour, rolled oats, baking soda, baking powder, powdered cinnamon, and salt in a large mixing basin. Blend well.

3. In a separate dish, thoroughly mix the unsweetened applesauce, almond milk, egg, vanilla extract, honey (or maple syrup).

4. Combine the wet and dry ingredients, mixing gently until blended. Take caution not to blend too much.

5. Gently incorporate the finely diced apple into the batter until it is mixed up completely.

6. Lightly mist a muffin tray or silicone muffin cups with nonstick spray.

7. Using a spoon, scoop out the batter and fill each muffin cup approximately 3/4 of the way.

8. To ensure enough air circulation, place the muffin cups in the air fryer basket, making sure they do not touch.

9. Bake the muffins for 12 to 15 minutes at 350°F/175°C, or until a toothpick is inserted into the middle of one and comes out clean.

10. Gently take the muffin cups out of the air fryer and let them rest for a few minutes in the cups before moving them to a wire rack to finish cooling.

11. Savor the muffins hot or at room temperature. Any leftovers can be kept in the fridge for up to a

week or to three days when stored in an airtight container.

Nutritional Information (per muffin, based on 8 muffins):

- **Calories: 150**
- **Protein: 3g**
- **Carbohydrates: 28g**
- **Dietary Fiber: 3g**
- **Sugars: 12g**
- **Total Fat: 3g**
- **Saturated Fat: 0.5g**
- **Sodium: 180mg**
- **Potassium: 120mg**

9. Quinoa Breakfast Bowls

Ingredients:

- 1 cup cooked quinoa
- 1/2 cup cherry tomatoes, halved
- 1/2 cup spinach leaves
- 1/2 avocado, diced
- 2 large eggs
- 1/4 cup feta cheese, crumbled (optional)
- 1/4 tsp garlic powder
- 1/4 tsp black pepper

- 1/8 tsp salt
- 1 tbsp olive oil
- Fresh parsley for garnish (optional)

Instructions:

1. For three minutes, preheat the air fryer to 350°F (175°C).
2. Combine the cherry tomatoes, salt, black pepper, garlic powder, and 1/2 tablespoon olive oil in a small bowl.
3. Put the cherry tomatoes in the air fryer basket and cook for five to seven minutes, or until they begin to soften and blister, at 350°F (175°C). 4. Add the remaining 1/2 tablespoon of olive oil to a pan and heat it over medium heat while the tomatoes are cooking.
5. Cook the spinach leaves in the pan for two to three minutes, or until they wilt. 6. Cook the eggs in a different little skillet according to your taste (scrambled, fried, or poached).
7. Take the tomatoes out of the air fryer and place them aside once they're done.
8. Split the cooked quinoa into two bowls to make the breakfast bowls.
9. Place the cooked eggs, avocado, roasted cherry tomatoes, and sautéed spinach on top of each bowl.
10. Garnish with fresh parsley and, if using, feta cheese.

11. Serve warm and enjoy.

.

Nutritional Information (per serving, based on 2 servings):

- **Calories: 350**
- **Protein: 14g**
- **Carbohydrates: 30g**
- **Dietary Fiber: 7g**
- **Sugars: 3g**
- **Total Fat: 20g**
- **Saturated Fat: 4g**
- **Sodium: 300mg**
- **Potassium: 700mg**

10. Air Fryer Chickpea Patties

Ingredients:

- 1 can (15 oz) chickpeas, drained and rinsed
- 1/2 cup rolled oats
- 1/4 cup chopped onion
- 1/4 cup chopped fresh parsley
- 2 cloves garlic, minced
- 1 large egg
- 1 tsp ground cumin
- 1 tsp ground coriander

- 1/2 tsp paprika
- 1/4 tsp salt
- 1/4 tsp black pepper
- 1 tbsp olive oil
- Non-stick spray

Instructions:

1. Place the chickpeas, rolled oats, minced garlic, diced onion, and parsley in a food processor. Pulse the mixture until it's well mixed but has some chunks remaining.

2. Fill the food processor with the egg, paprika, ground coriander, ground cumin, ground coriander, salt, and black pepper. Repeatedly pulse until all components are well combined.

3. Pour the mixture into a big basin and shape it into patties, each with a diameter of two to three inches. About 6–8 patties should be produced.

4. For three minutes, preheat the air fryer to 375°F (190°C).

5. To avoid sticking, lightly mist the air fryer basket with non-stick spray. 6. To make the patties crispier, lightly coat each one with olive oil.

7. Make sure the patties are not in contact with one another by placing them in the air fryer basket in a single layer.

8. Air fry the chickpea patties for 10 to 12 minutes at 375°F (190°C), turning them halfway through, or

until they are crispy and golden brown on both sides.

9. Before serving, carefully take the patties out of the air fryer and allow them to cool for a few minutes.

10. You may serve the heated chickpea patties over a salad or sandwich, or you can serve them with your preferred dipping sauce.

Nutritional Information (per patty, based on 8 patties):

- **Calories: 120**
- **Protein: 5g**
- **Carbohydrates: 18g**
- **Dietary Fiber: 4g**
- **Sugars: 1g**
- **Total Fat: 3g**
- **Saturated Fat: 0.5g**
- **Sodium: 200mg**
- **Potassium: 150mg**

11. Baked Pears with Cinnamon

Ingredients:

- 2 ripe pears

- 1 tablespoon honey or maple syrup (optional, check with your dietitian)
- 1 teaspoon ground cinnamon
- 1/4 teaspoon ground nutmeg
- 1/4 teaspoon ground ginger
- 1/4 cup water
- Fresh mint leaves for garnish (optional)

Instructions:

1. Give the pears a good wash.
2. Using a spoon or melon baller, cut the pears in half and remove the seeds and core.
3. Combine the ginger, nutmeg, and ground cinnamon in a small bowl.
4. Evenly distribute the spice mixture over the pears' sliced sides.
5. If using, drizzle maple syrup or honey over the pears.
6. Set your air fryer's temperature for three to five minutes at 350°F (175°C).
7. Put the pear halves, cut side up, in the air fryer basket.
8. To keep the pears from drying out, add 1/4 cup of water to the bottom of the air fryer basket, right under the pears.
9. Cook the pears for 12 to 15 minutes, or until they are soft and browned.

10. Using tongs, carefully take the pears out of the air fryer.

11. Before serving, let them cool somewhat.

12. If preferred, garnish with fresh mint leaves.

Nutritional Information (per serving, based on 1 pear half):

- **Calories: 60**
- **Protein: 0.5g**
- **Carbohydrates: 16g**
- **Dietary Fiber: 3g**
- **Sugars: 10g (varies if using honey or maple syrup)**
- **Fat: 0g**
- **Sodium: 0mg**
- **Potassium: 150mg**
- **Phosphorus: 10mg**

12. Zucchini and Carrot Breakfast Fritters

Ingredients:

- 1 medium zucchini, grated
- 1 medium carrot, grated

- 1/4 cup whole wheat flour
- 1 egg
- 1/4 teaspoon salt (optional, check with your dietitian)
- 1/4 teaspoon ground black pepper
- 1/4 teaspoon garlic powder
- 1/4 teaspoon onion powder
- 1 tablespoon fresh parsley, chopped (optional)
- Olive oil spray

Instructions:

1. Using a box grater, grate the carrot and zucchini.
2. Squeeze off as much moisture from the grated zucchini using a clean kitchen towel.
3. Combine the grated carrot and zucchini, whole wheat flour, egg, salt, pepper, onion powder, garlic powder, and chopped parsley (if using) in a big bowl. Blend thoroughly until everything is properly integrated.
4. Set your air fryer's temperature for three to five minutes at 375°F (190°C).
5. Shape the mixture into little fritters with a diameter of two to three inches, then gently press them flat.
6. To keep the air fryer basket from sticking, lightly mist it with olive oil spray.

7. To ensure consistent cooking, arrange the fritters in the air fryer basket in a single layer, allowing space between them.

8. Gently mist the fritters' tops with olive oil spray.

9. Cook for 8 to 10 minutes, then turn the fritters over and continue cooking for 5 to 7 more minutes, or until crispy and golden brown.

10. Using tongs or a spatula, carefully remove the fritters from the air fryer.

11. Before serving, let them cool somewhat.

Nutritional Information (per fritter):

- **Calories: 45**
- **Protein: 2g**
- **Carbohydrates: 6g**
- **Dietary Fiber: 1g**
- **Sugars: 1g**
- **Fat: 1g**
- **Sodium: 45mg (varies with salt content)**
- **Potassium: 150mg**
- **Phosphorus: 25mg**

CHAPTER FOUR: MOUTHWATERING KIDNEY TRANSPLANT AIR FRYER LUNCH RECIPES

Welcome to the Kidney Transplant Air Fryer Diet Cookbook's section on lunch recipes. Here are some tasty, healthful, and kidney-friendly lunch options that you can quickly make with an air fryer. These recipes emphasize lean meats, nutritious grains, and fresh veggies in an effort to maintain your health following a transplant. Savor these delicious meals that will provide you with energy and satisfaction all day long.

1. Air Fryer Quinoa-Stuffed Bell Peppers

Ingredients:

- 4 medium bell peppers (any color)
- 1 cup cooked quinoa
- 1/2 cup canned black beans, rinsed and drained
- 1/2 cup corn kernels (fresh, frozen, or canned)
- 1 small onion, finely chopped
- 1 clove garlic, minced
- 1 teaspoon ground cumin
- 1 teaspoon chili powder
- 1/2 teaspoon paprika
- 1/4 teaspoon salt (optional, check with your dietitian)
- 1/4 teaspoon ground black pepper
- 1/2 cup shredded low-fat cheese (optional, check with your dietitian)
- Fresh cilantro for garnish (optional)
- Olive oil spray

Instructions:

1. Slice off the bell peppers' tops, then take out the seeds and membranes. Put aside.
2. Put the cooked quinoa, black beans, corn, chopped onion, minced garlic, ground cumin, paprika, chili powder, salt, and black pepper in a big bowl. Blend thoroughly until everything is properly integrated.

3. Gently press down to firmly put the quinoa mixture inside each bell pepper.

4. Top each filled pepper with a little quantity of cheese, if using.

5. Set your air fryer's temperature for three to five minutes at 360°F (180°C).

6. To keep the air fryer basket from sticking, lightly mist it with olive oil spray.

7. Holding the filled bell peppers upright, place them in the air fryer basket. The number of batches you need to cook them in will depend on how big your air fryer is.

8. Simmer for ten to fifteen minutes, or until the filling is well cooked and the peppers are soft. If cheese is being used, it must be bubbling and melted.

9. Using tongs, carefully take the bell peppers out of the air fryer.

10. Before serving, allow them to cool somewhat.

11. If preferred, garnish with fresh cilantro.

Nutritional Information (per stuffed pepper, without cheese):

- **Calories: 150**
- **Protein: 5g**
- **Carbohydrates: 30g**
- **Dietary Fiber: 6g**
- **Sugars: 5g**

- **Fat: 1.5g**
- **Sodium: 120mg (varies with salt content)**
- **Potassium: 500mg**
- **Phosphorus: 100mg**

2. Chickpea and Veggie Patties

Ingredients:

- 1 can (15 oz) chickpeas, rinsed and drained
- 1 small carrot, grated
- 1 small zucchini, grated and excess water squeezed out
- 1/4 cup finely chopped red bell pepper
- 1/4 cup finely chopped red onion
- 1 clove garlic, minced
- 1/4 cup whole wheat breadcrumbs
- 1 egg
- 1 teaspoon ground cumin
- 1/2 teaspoon ground coriander
- 1/4 teaspoon ground black pepper
- 1/4 teaspoon salt (optional, check with your dietitian)
- 1 tablespoon fresh parsley or cilantro, chopped (optional)
- Olive oil spray

Instructions:

1. Using a fork or potato masher, mash the chickpeas in a big basin until they are mostly smooth but still have some chunks.

2. To the mashed chickpeas, add the shredded carrot, grated zucchini, diced red bell pepper, chopped red onion, and minced garlic. Blend well.

3. Fully incorporate the ground cumin, ground coriander, black pepper, salt, egg, and chopped parsley or cilantro (if using) with the whole wheat breadcrumbs.

4. Shape the mixture into little patties that are 1/2 inch thick and have a diameter of two to three inches.

5. Take around three to five minutes to preheat your air fryer to 375°F (190°C).

6. To keep the air fryer basket from sticking, lightly mist it with olive oil spray.

7. To ensure equal cooking, arrange the patties in the air fryer basket in a single layer with room between them.

8. Gently mist the patties' tops with olive oil spray.

9. Cook for 10 to 12 minutes, turning the patties halfway through, or until the outsides are crispy and golden brown.

10. Using tongs or a spatula, carefully remove the patties from the air fryer.

11. Before serving, let them cool somewhat.

Nutritional Information (per patty):

- **Calories: 80**
- **Protein: 3g**
- **Carbohydrates: 12g**
- **Dietary Fiber: 3g**
- **Sugars: 2g**
- **Fat: 2g**
- **Sodium: 100mg (varies with salt content)**
- **Potassium: 150mg**
- **Phosphorus: 50mg**

3. Air Fryer Tofu and Veggie Stir-Fry

Ingredients:

- 1 block (14 oz) firm tofu, drained and pressed
- 1 small zucchini, sliced
- 1 small red bell pepper, sliced
- 1 small yellow bell pepper, sliced
- 1 cup broccoli florets
- 1 small carrot, thinly sliced
- 1 tablespoon olive oil
- 2 tablespoons low-sodium soy sauce
- 1 tablespoon rice vinegar
- 1 teaspoon garlic powder

- 1 teaspoon onion powder
- 1/4 teaspoon ground black pepper
- 1/4 teaspoon ground ginger
- 1 teaspoon sesame seeds (optional)
- Fresh cilantro or green onions for garnish (optional)

Instructions:

1. Create 1-inch cubes out of the pressed tofu.

2. Put the tofu cubes in a big bowl together with 1/2 teaspoon of onion powder, 1/4 tablespoon of low-sodium soy sauce, and 1 tablespoon of olive oil. For uniform coating of the tofu, lightly toss.

3. Set your air fryer's temperature for three to five minutes at 375°F (190°C).

4. To keep the air fryer basket from sticking, lightly mist it with olive oil spray.

5. Arrange the tofu cubes in a single layer within the air fryer basket. Shake the basket halfway through and cook for 10 to 12 minutes, or until the tofu is crispy and golden brown.

6. Prepare the veggies while the tofu is cooking. Sliced carrots, broccoli florets, red and yellow bell peppers, and zucchini should all be combined in a big bowl.

7. Combine the veggies with 1 tablespoon of low-sodium soy sauce, 1 tablespoon rice vinegar, 1/2 teaspoon each of onion and garlic powder,

powdered black pepper, and ground ginger. For an even coat, toss.

8. Carefully take the cooked tofu out of the air fryer and place it aside.

9. Put the veggies in the air fryer basket and cook for 10 to 12 minutes, shaking the basket halfway through, at 375°F (190°C), or until the vegetables are soft and just beginning to brown.

10. To fully heat everything through, return the tofu and veggies to the air fryer basket and cook for a further two to three minutes.

11. Carefully take the veggies and tofu out of the air fryer and place them on a platter for serving.

12. If preferred, add some sesame seeds and fresh cilantro or green onions as garnish.

Nutritional Information (per serving):

- **Calories: 180**
- **Protein: 10g**
- **Carbohydrates: 14g**
- **Dietary Fiber: 4g**
- **Sugars: 4g**
- **Fat: 10g**
- **Sodium: 250mg (varies with soy sauce content)**
- **Potassium: 350mg**
- **Phosphorus: 120mg**

4. Sweet Potato and Black Bean Tacos

Ingredients:

- 2 medium sweet potatoes, peeled and diced
- 1 can (15 oz) black beans, rinsed and drained
- 1 small red onion, diced
- 1 small red bell pepper, diced
- 1 tablespoon olive oil
- 1 teaspoon ground cumin
- 1/2 teaspoon chili powder
- 1/2 teaspoon paprika
- 1/4 teaspoon ground black pepper
- 1/4 teaspoon salt (optional, check with your dietitian)
- 8 small corn tortillas
- Fresh cilantro for garnish (optional)
- Lime wedges for serving (optional)

Instructions:

1. Set your air fryer's temperature for three to five minutes at 375°F (190°C).
2. Place the diced sweet potatoes in a big basin and toss them until they are uniformly coated with olive oil, ground cumin, chili powder, paprika, black pepper, and salt (if using).

3. To keep the air fryer basket from sticking, lightly mist it with olive oil spray.

4. Arrange the seasoned sweet potatoes in a single layer within the air fryer basket. Sweet potatoes should be cooked for 15 to 20 minutes, shaking the basket halfway through, or until they are soft and beginning to crisp up.

5. In a medium-sized dish, mix the diced red onion, diced red bell pepper, and black beans while the sweet potatoes are cooking. Put aside.

6. Carefully take the sweet potatoes out of the air fryer and combine them with the black bean mixture. Gently toss to mix.

7. Use the air fryer to reheat the corn tortillas for one to two minutes, or until they are soft and malleable.

8. Spoon the black bean and sweet potato mixture onto each tortilla to assemble the tacos.

9. If preferred, garnish with fresh cilantro and serve with lime wedges.

Nutritional Information (per taco):

- **Calories: 120**
- **Protein: 3g**
- **Carbohydrates: 23g**
- **Dietary Fiber: 5g**
- **Sugars: 3g**
- **Fat: 3g**

- **Sodium: 150mg (varies with salt content)**
- **Potassium: 350mg**
- **Phosphorus: 60mg**

5. Cauliflower and Lentil Rice Bowls

Ingredients:

- 1 medium head of cauliflower, cut into florets
- 1 cup cooked lentils (brown or green)
- 1 cup cooked brown rice
- 1 small red bell pepper, diced
- 1 small cucumber, diced
- 1 small carrot, grated
- 1/4 cup red onion, finely chopped
- 1 tablespoon olive oil
- 1 teaspoon ground cumin
- 1/2 teaspoon smoked paprika
- 1/4 teaspoon ground black pepper
- 1/4 teaspoon salt (optional, check with your dietitian)
- 1 tablespoon fresh parsley or cilantro, chopped (optional)
- Lemon wedges for serving (optional)

Instructions:

1. Set your air fryer's temperature for three to five minutes at 375°F (190°C).

2. Place the cauliflower florets in a big basin and toss them until they are uniformly coated with olive oil, smoked paprika, ground cumin, black pepper, and salt (if using).

3. To keep the air fryer basket from sticking, lightly mist it with olive oil spray.

4. Arrange the seasoned cauliflower florets in a single layer within the air fryer basket. Cook, shaking the basket halfway through, until the cauliflower is soft and beginning to crisp up, 12 to 15 minutes.

5. Prepare the remaining ingredients while the cauliflower cooks. The cooked lentils, cooked brown rice, sliced cucumber, diced bell pepper, shredded carrot, and chopped red onion should all be combined in a big bowl. Gently toss to mix.

6. Carefully take the cauliflower out of the air fryer and add it to the bowl containing the rice and lentil mixture. Gently toss to mix.

7. Transfer the mixture into dishes and, if preferred, top with cilantro or fresh parsley.

8. For an additional taste explosion, serve with lemon slices on the side.

Nutritional Information (per serving, based on 4 servings):

- **Calories: 220**
- **Protein: 8g**
- **Carbohydrates: 35g**
- **Dietary Fiber: 10g**
- **Sugars: 5g**
- **Fat: 5g**
- **Sodium: 150mg (varies with salt content)**
- **Potassium: 600mg**
- **Phosphorus: 150mg**

6. Air Fryer Falafel with Tabouli

Ingredients:

For the Falafel:

- 1 can (15 oz) chickpeas, rinsed and drained
- 1/4 cup chopped fresh parsley
- 1/4 cup chopped fresh cilantro
- 1 small onion, finely chopped
- 2 cloves garlic, minced
- 1 teaspoon ground cumin
- 1 teaspoon ground coriander
- 1/2 teaspoon ground black pepper
- 1/2 teaspoon salt (optional, check with your dietitian)
- 1/4 teaspoon baking soda
- 1 tablespoon whole wheat flour

- 1 tablespoon olive oil
- Olive oil spray

For the Tabouli:

- 1/2 cup bulgur wheat
- 1 cup boiling water
- 1 cup finely chopped fresh parsley
- 1/2 cup finely chopped fresh mint
- 1/2 cup finely chopped tomato
- 1/4 cup finely chopped cucumber
- 1/4 cup finely chopped red onion
- 1/4 cup fresh lemon juice
- 2 tablespoons olive oil
- 1/4 teaspoon ground black pepper
- 1/4 teaspoon salt (optional, check with your dietitian)

Instructions:

Prepare the Falafel:

1. Put the chickpeas, black pepper, cumin, coriander, onion, garlic, parsley, cilantro, and salt (if using) in a food processor. Pulse the mixture until it's thoroughly blended and coarse.
2. Pour the liquid into a basin and whisk in the whole wheat flour and baking soda. Blend the items thoroughly until they are properly blended.

3. Create little, 1.5-inch-diameter balls out of the mixture, then gently press them down to resemble patties.

4. Set your air fryer's temperature for three to five minutes at 375°F (190°C).

5. To keep the air fryer basket from sticking, lightly mist it with olive oil spray.

6. To ensure equal cooking, arrange the falafel patties in the air fryer basket in a single layer, allowing space between them. Apply a little layer of olive oil spray to the tops.

7. Cook the falafel for 12 to 15 minutes, turning them halfway through, or until they are crispy and golden brown.

8. Using tongs or a spatula, carefully take the falafel out of the air fryer and place it aside.

Prepare the Tabouli:

1. Transfer the bulgur wheat to a big bowl and cover it with the boiling water. Once the bulgur is soft and has absorbed the water, cover and let it sit for 15 to 20 minutes.

2. Use a fork to fluff the bulgur and let it cool slightly.

3. Top the bulgur with the chopped red onion, tomato, cucumber, mint, and parsley. Blend well.

4. Combine the lemon juice, olive oil, salt (if using), and black pepper in a small bowl. After pouring the dressing over the tabouli, toss to ensure uniform coating.

Assemble and Serve:

1. Present the tabouli and falafel patties side by side. If preferred, garnish with extra fresh herbs and slices of lemon.

Nutritional Information (per serving, based on 4 servings):

Falafel:

- **Calories: 180**
- **Protein: 6g**
- **Carbohydrates: 22g**
- **Dietary Fiber: 5g**
- **Sugars: 2g**
- **Fat: 7g**
- **Sodium: 200mg (varies with salt content)**
- **Potassium: 250mg**
- **Phosphorus: 100mg**

Tabouli:

- **Calories: 120**

- **Protein: 2g**
- **Carbohydrates: 18g**
- **Dietary Fiber: 4g**
- **Sugars: 2g**
- **Fat: 5g**
- **Sodium: 100mg (varies with salt content)**
- **Potassium: 300mg**
- **Phosphorus: 40mg**

7. Brussels Sprouts and Quinoa Salad

Ingredients:

- 1 cup quinoa, rinsed
- 2 cups water
- 1 pound Brussels sprouts, trimmed and halved
- 1 tablespoon olive oil
- 1 small red onion, thinly sliced
- 1/2 cup dried cranberries
- 1/4 cup chopped walnuts (optional, check with your dietitian)
- 1/4 cup fresh parsley, chopped
- 1/4 teaspoon salt (optional, check with your dietitian)
- 1/4 teaspoon ground black pepper

For the Dressing:

- 1/4 cup olive oil
- 2 tablespoons apple cider vinegar
- 1 tablespoon Dijon mustard
- 1 tablespoon honey or maple syrup (optional, check with your dietitian)
- 1/4 teaspoon ground black pepper
- 1/4 teaspoon salt (optional, check with your dietitian)

Instructions:

1. In a medium saucepan, bring two cups of water to a boil before cooking the quinoa. Add the rinsed quinoa, lower the heat to low, cover, and simmer for about 15 minutes until the quinoa is soft and the water has been absorbed. Using a fork, fluff and set aside to cool.

2. Set your air fryer's temperature for three to five minutes at 375°F (190°C).

3. Combine the halved Brussels sprouts, 1 tablespoon olive oil, black pepper, and salt (if needed) in a big dish.

4. To keep the air fryer basket from sticking, lightly mist it with olive oil spray.

5. Arrange the Brussels sprouts in a single layer within the air fryer basket. Shake the basket halfway through cooking the Brussels sprouts for 12

to 15 minutes, or until they are crispy and golden brown.

6. Put the cooked quinoa, chopped parsley, dried cranberries, roasted Brussels sprouts, sliced red onion, and chopped walnuts (if using) in a big mixing dish.

7. To make the dressing, combine the olive oil, Dijon mustard, apple cider vinegar, honey or maple syrup (if desired), black pepper, and salt (if applicable) in a small bowl.

8. Drizzle the Brussels sprouts and quinoa mixture with the dressing. Make sure everything is uniformly covered by giving it a good toss.

9. You may serve the salad room temperature or heated.

Nutritional Information (per serving, based on 4 servings):

- **Calories: 320**
- **Protein: 7g**
- **Carbohydrates: 38g**
- **Dietary Fiber: 7g**
- **Sugars: 10g (varies if using honey or maple syrup)**
- **Fat: 16g**
- **Sodium: 200mg (varies with salt content)**
- **Potassium: 500mg**
- **Phosphorus: 150mg**

8. Stuffed Zucchini Boats

Ingredients:

- 4 medium zucchini
- 1 cup cooked quinoa
- 1/2 cup canned black beans, rinsed and drained
- 1 small red bell pepper, diced
- 1 small red onion, diced
- 1 clove garlic, minced
- 1 teaspoon ground cumin
- 1/2 teaspoon chili powder
- 1/4 teaspoon paprika
- 1/4 teaspoon ground black pepper
- 1/4 teaspoon salt (optional, check with your dietitian)
- 1/2 cup shredded low-fat cheese (optional, check with your dietitian)
- Fresh cilantro for garnish (optional)
- Olive oil spray

Instructions:

1. Set your air fryer's temperature for three to five minutes at 375°F (190°C).
2. After giving the zucchini a good wash, split them in half lengthwise. Scoop out the seeds and flesh

using a spoon to form a hollow boat. Spooned flesh should be set away.

3. Insert the zucchini boats into the air fryer basket after giving them a quick mist of olive oil spray. Cook for five minutes to gently tenderize.

4. Chop the scooped zucchini flesh and set it aside while the zucchini boats cook.

5. Combine the cooked quinoa, black beans, diced red onion, diced bell pepper, minced garlic, sliced zucchini flesh, ground cumin, paprika, chili powder, black pepper, and salt (if used) in a medium-sized bowl. Blend thoroughly until everything is properly integrated.

6. Take the zucchini boats out of the air fryer and carefully put the filling into them by pressing down on the zucchini boats.

7. Top each filled zucchini boat with a little quantity of cheese, if using.

8. Reposition the filled zucchini boats in a single layer within the air fryer basket. Simmer for a further 10 to 12 minutes, or until the filling is well cooked and the zucchini are soft. If cheese is being used, it must be bubbling and melted.

9. Using tongs, carefully take the zucchini boats out of the air fryer.

10. Before serving, allow them to cool somewhat.

11. If preferred, garnish with fresh cilantro.

Nutritional Information (per stuffed zucchini boat):

- **Calories: 150**
- **Protein: 5g**
- **Carbohydrates: 24g**
- **Dietary Fiber: 5g**
- **Sugars: 6g**
- **Fat: 3g**
- **Sodium: 200mg (varies with salt content)**
- **Potassium: 500mg**
- **Phosphorus: 100mg**

9. Air Fryer Eggplant Parmesan

Ingredients:

- 1 large eggplant, sliced into 1/4-inch thick rounds
- 1 teaspoon salt (optional, check with your dietitian)
- 1 cup whole wheat breadcrumbs
- 1/2 cup grated Parmesan cheese
- 1 teaspoon Italian seasoning
- 1/2 teaspoon garlic powder
- 1/2 teaspoon onion powder
- 1/4 teaspoon ground black pepper
- 2 eggs, beaten
- 1 cup marinara sauce (low sodium)

- 1 cup shredded mozzarella cheese (optional, check with your dietitian)
- Fresh basil for garnish (optional)
- Olive oil spray

Instructions:

1. Arrange the eggplant slices on a large baking sheet and, if desired, season with salt. After allowing them to sit for ten to fifteen minutes to absorb moisture, blot them dry with paper towels.

2. Transfer the whole wheat breadcrumbs, grated Parmesan cheese, Italian seasoning, onion and garlic powders, and black pepper into a shallow basin.

3. Beat the eggs in a different, small basin.

4. Set your air fryer's temperature for three to five minutes at 375°F (190°C).

5. Coat each eggplant slice in the breadcrumb mixture after dipping it into the beaten eggs, gently pressing to adhere.

6. To keep the air fryer basket from sticking, lightly mist it with olive oil spray.

7. To ensure consistent cooking, arrange the breaded eggplant slices in the air fryer basket in a single layer, with space between them. Apply a little layer of olive oil spray to the tops.

8. Cook the eggplant for 10 to 12 minutes, turning it halfway through, or until it's crispy and golden brown.

9. Cover the bottom of a baking dish or plate that fits inside your air fryer with a thin coating of marinara sauce.

10. Cover the marinara sauce with a layer of cooked eggplant pieces. Drizzle the eggplant with more marinara sauce and, if desired, top with shredded mozzarella cheese.

11. Continue layering, then finish with a dollop of mozzarella cheese and marinara sauce.

12. Put the stacked eggplant back in the air fryer and cook it for five to seven minutes, or until the cheese is bubbling and melted, at 350°F (175°C).

13. Take the eggplant Parmesan out of the air fryer with care.

14. If preferred, garnish with fresh basil.

Nutritional Information (per serving, based on 4 servings):

- **Calories: 220**
- **Protein: 10g**
- **Carbohydrates: 24g**
- **Dietary Fiber: 7g**
- **Sugars: 9g**
- **Fat: 9g**

- **Sodium: 300mg (varies with salt and marinara sauce content)**
- **Potassium: 600mg**
- **Phosphorus: 150mg**

10. Spicy Air Fryer Cauliflower Tacos

Ingredients:

- 1 medium head of cauliflower, cut into florets
- 1 tablespoon olive oil
- 1 teaspoon chili powder
- 1 teaspoon smoked paprika
- 1/2 teaspoon ground cumin
- 1/4 teaspoon garlic powder
- 1/4 teaspoon onion powder
- 1/4 teaspoon ground black pepper
- 1/4 teaspoon salt (optional, check with your dietitian)
- 8 small corn tortillas
- 1/2 cup shredded red cabbage
- 1 small avocado, sliced
- 1/4 cup chopped fresh cilantro
- Lime wedges for serving

For the Spicy Sauce:

- 1/4 cup plain Greek yogurt (or a dairy-free alternative)
- 1 tablespoon hot sauce (adjust to taste)
- 1 tablespoon lime juice
- 1/4 teaspoon garlic powder
- 1/4 teaspoon smoked paprika

Instructions:

1. Set your air fryer's temperature for three to five minutes at 375°F (190°C).
2. Place the cauliflower florets in a big basin and toss them until they are uniformly coated with olive oil, ground cumin, smoked paprika, chili powder, onion powder, garlic powder, black pepper, and salt (if using).
3. To keep the air fryer basket from sticking, lightly mist it with olive oil spray.
4. Arrange the seasoned cauliflower florets in a single layer within the air fryer basket. Cook, shaking the basket halfway through, until the cauliflower is soft and beginning to crisp up, 12 to 15 minutes.
5. In a separate bowl, mix together the Greek yogurt, hot sauce, lime juice, garlic powder, and smoked paprika to make the spicy sauce while the cauliflower cooks. To taste, adjust the spicy sauce.

6. Use the air fryer to reheat the corn tortillas for one to two minutes, or until they are malleable and soft.

7. Put some of the cooked cauliflower on each tortilla to assemble the tacos.

8. Add chopped cilantro, avocado slices, and shredded red cabbage on top.

9. Top each taco with a drizzle of the hot sauce.

10. For an additional taste boost, serve with lime wedges on the side.

Nutritional Information (per taco, based on 8 tacos):

- **Calories: 130**
- **Protein: 3g**
- **Carbohydrates: 19g**
- **Dietary Fiber: 5g**
- **Sugars: 2g**
- **Fat: 6g**
- **Sodium: 200mg (varies with salt content and hot sauce)**
- **Potassium: 350mg**
- **Phosphorus: 50mg**

11. Air Fryer Tempeh and Veggie Skewers

Ingredients:

- 1 block (8 oz) tempeh, cut into 1-inch cubes
- 1 red bell pepper, cut into 1-inch pieces
- 1 yellow bell pepper, cut into 1-inch pieces
- 1 small zucchini, sliced into 1/2-inch rounds
- 1 small red onion, cut into wedges
- 1 cup cherry tomatoes
- Olive oil spray

For the Marinade:

- 2 tablespoons low-sodium soy sauce
- 1 tablespoon olive oil
- 1 tablespoon maple syrup or honey (optional, check with your dietitian)
- 1 tablespoon apple cider vinegar
- 1 teaspoon garlic powder
- 1 teaspoon smoked paprika
- 1/2 teaspoon ground cumin
- 1/4 teaspoon ground black pepper

Instructions:

1. Combine all the marinade ingredients (olive oil, low-sodium soy sauce, smoked paprika, ground cumin, apple cider vinegar, maple syrup, or honey, if using) in a small bowl.

2. Transfer the marinade to a shallow dish and cover the tempeh cubes. For an even coat, toss. Give it a minimum of 30 minutes to marinate, or up to 2 hours for maximum flavor.

3. Chop the red and yellow bell peppers into 1-inch chunks, slice the zucchini into 1/2-inch rounds, and cut the red onion into wedges while the tempeh is marinating.

4. Set your air fryer's temperature for three to five minutes at 375°F (190°C).

5. Thread the bell peppers, zucchini, red onion, cherry tomatoes, and marinated tempeh and prepared veggies onto skewers in alternate order.

6. To keep the air fryer basket from sticking, lightly mist it with olive oil spray.

7. Arrange the skewers in a single layer within the air fryer basket. The number of batches you need to cook them in will depend on how big your air fryer is.

8. Cook the skewers for 10 to 12 minutes, turning them halfway through, or until the veggies are soft and the tempeh is golden brown.

9. Using tongs, carefully take the skewers out of the air fryer.

10. Before serving, allow them to cool somewhat.

Nutritional Information (per skewer, based on 8 skewers):

- **Calories: 100**
- **Protein: 6g**
- **Carbohydrates: 10g**
- **Dietary Fiber: 3g**
- **Sugars: 5g (varies if using maple syrup or honey)**
- **Fat: 4g**
- **Sodium: 200mg (varies with soy sauce content)**
- **Potassium: 350mg**
- **Phosphorus: 80mg**

12. Air Fryer Kale and Chickpea Salad

Ingredients:

- 1 bunch of kale, washed and torn into bite-sized pieces (stems removed)
- 1 can (15 oz) chickpeas, rinsed and drained
- 1 tablespoon olive oil
- 1 teaspoon smoked paprika
- 1/2 teaspoon garlic powder
- 1/2 teaspoon ground cumin
- 1/4 teaspoon ground black pepper
- 1/4 teaspoon salt (optional, check with your dietitian)
- 1/2 cup cherry tomatoes, halved

- 1/4 cup red onion, thinly sliced
- 1/4 cup shredded carrots
- 1/4 cup sunflower seeds (optional, check with your dietitian)
- Lemon wedges for serving

For the Dressing:

- 3 tablespoons olive oil
- 2 tablespoons lemon juice
- 1 teaspoon Dijon mustard
- 1 teaspoon honey or maple syrup (optional, check with your dietitian)
- 1/4 teaspoon ground black pepper
- 1/4 teaspoon salt (optional, check with your dietitian)

Instructions:

1. Set your air fryer's temperature for three to five minutes at 375°F (190°C).
2. Place the chickpeas in a big basin and toss them until they are uniformly coated with 1/2 tablespoon olive oil, smoked paprika, garlic powder, ground cumin, black pepper, and salt (if using).
3. To keep the air fryer basket from sticking, lightly mist it with olive oil spray.
4. Spread out in a single layer within the air fryer basket the seasoned chickpeas. Shake the basket

halfway through cooking the chickpeas for 10 to 12 minutes, or until they are crispy and golden brown.

5. Toss the kale pieces with the remaining 1/2 tablespoon of olive oil while the chickpeas are cooking. To help tenderize the kale, give it a gentle massage.

6. Take the chickpeas out of the air fryer and place them aside once they're done.

7. Put the kale in a single layer within the air fryer basket. Shake the basket halfway through cooking the kale for 4–6 minutes, or until it becomes crispy but not charred.

8. Combine the dressing ingredients in a small bowl, whisking in the olive oil, lemon juice, Dijon mustard, black pepper, honey or maple syrup (if used), and salt (if using).

9. Put the roasted chickpeas, cherry tomatoes, red onion, shredded carrots, crispy kale, and sunflower seeds (if using) in a big mixing bowl.

10. Pour the dressing over the salad and toss to coat evenly.

11. To add even more flavor, serve the salad right away with lemon wedges on the side.

Nutritional Information (per serving, based on 4 servings):

- **Calories: 220**
- **Protein: 5g**

- Carbohydrates: 19g
- Dietary Fiber: 6g
- Sugars: 5g (varies if using honey or maple syrup)
- Fat: 14g
- Sodium: 200mg (varies with salt content)
- Potassium: 600mg
- Phosphorus: 100mg

CHAPTER FIVE: DELICIOUS KIDNEY TRANSPLANT AIR FRYER DINNER RECIPES

The Kidney Transplant Air Fryer Diet Cookbook's supper recipe section is here. This is where you may find a variety of tasty and filling dinner alternatives designed to promote your health after transplant surgery. Air fryers make it easy to cook nutritious ingredients like fresh veggies, whole grains, and lean meats for these dishes. Suppertimes should be enjoyable and fulfilling, ending the day on a pleasant note.

1. Air Fryer Lentil-Stuffed Portobello Mushrooms

Ingredients:

- 4 large portobello mushrooms, stems removed and gills scraped out
- 1 cup cooked lentils
- 1 small onion, finely chopped
- 1 small red bell pepper, finely chopped
- 1 clove garlic, minced
- 1/4 cup whole wheat breadcrumbs
- 1/4 cup grated Parmesan cheese (optional, check with your dietitian)
- 1 tablespoon fresh parsley, chopped (optional)
- 1 tablespoon olive oil
- 1 teaspoon Italian seasoning
- 1/4 teaspoon ground black pepper
- 1/4 teaspoon salt (optional, check with your dietitian)
- Olive oil spray

Instructions:

1. Set your air fryer's temperature for three to five minutes at 375°F (190°C).
2. Heat the olive oil in a big skillet over medium heat. Add the minced garlic, red bell pepper, and diced onion. Sauté for approximately five minutes, or until the veggies are tender.
3. Fill the skillet with the cooked lentils, Italian spice, black pepper, and salt (if using). After combining, cook for a further two to three minutes. Take off the heat.

4. Add the grated Parmesan cheese (if using) and whole wheat breadcrumbs to the lentil mixture. Blend thoroughly until everything is properly integrated.

5. Lightly mist both sides of the portobello mushroom caps with olive oil spray.

6. Spoon the lentil mixture into each mushroom cap, lightly pushing to compact the filling.

7. Arrange the filled mushrooms in a single layer within the air fryer basket. The number of batches you need to cook them in will depend on how big your air fryer is.

8. Cook for ten to twelve minutes, or until the filling is well cooked and has a hint of crunch on top, and the mushrooms are soft.

9. Using tongs, carefully take the stuffed mushrooms out of the air fryer.

10. Before serving, allow them to cool somewhat.

11. If preferred, garnish with fresh parsley.

Nutritional Information (per stuffed mushroom, based on 4 servings):

- **Calories: 180**
- **Protein: 9g**
- **Carbohydrates: 23g**
- **Dietary Fiber: 7g**
- **Sugars: 5g**
- **Fat: 6g**

- **Sodium: 220mg (varies with salt and cheese content)**
- **Potassium: 700mg**
- **Phosphorus: 140mg**

2. Crispy Air Fryer Tofu with Brown Rice and Veggies

Ingredients:

- 1 block (14 oz) firm tofu, drained and pressed
- 2 tablespoons low-sodium soy sauce
- 1 tablespoon olive oil
- 1 teaspoon garlic powder
- 1 teaspoon smoked paprika
- 1/4 teaspoon ground black pepper
- 1 cup cooked brown rice
- 1 cup broccoli florets
- 1 red bell pepper, sliced
- 1 small carrot, thinly sliced
- 1/2 cup snap peas
- Olive oil spray

For the Sauce:

- 2 tablespoons low-sodium soy sauce
- 1 tablespoon rice vinegar

- 1 teaspoon honey or maple syrup (optional, check with your dietitian)
- 1 teaspoon sesame oil
- 1/2 teaspoon ground ginger

Instructions:

1. Set your air fryer's temperature for three to five minutes at 375°F (190°C).
2. Create 1-inch cubes out of the pressed tofu.
3. Place the tofu cubes, 2 tablespoons of low-sodium soy sauce, olive oil, smoked paprika, black pepper, and garlic powder in a big bowl. For uniform coating of the tofu, lightly toss.
4. To keep the air fryer basket from sticking, lightly mist it with olive oil spray.
5. Arrange the tofu cubes in a single layer within the air fryer basket. Shake the basket halfway through and cook for 12 to 15 minutes, or until the tofu is crispy and golden brown.
6. Prepare the veggies while the tofu is cooking. Toss the broccoli florets, carrot slices, snap peas, and sliced red bell pepper in a separate bowl and lightly mist with olive oil spray.
7. Take the tofu out of the air fryer and place it aside once it's finished.
8. Put the veggies in the air fryer basket and cook for 8 to 10 minutes, shaking the basket halfway

through, at 375°F (190°C), or until the vegetables are soft and just beginning to brown.

9. Make the sauce while the veggies are cooking. Combine 2 teaspoons of low-sodium soy sauce, rice vinegar, ground ginger, honey or maple syrup (if desired), and sesame oil in a small bowl.

10. Transfer the cooked brown rice, air-fried tofu, and air-fried veggies into a large mixing dish. Pour the sauce over the mixture, tossing to ensure uniform coating.

11. Serve the crispy tofu and vegetable combination with brown rice.

Nutritional Information (per serving, based on 4 servings):

- **Calories: 300**
- **Protein: 12g**
- **Carbohydrates: 38g**
- **Dietary Fiber: 6g**
- **Sugars: 5g (varies if using honey or maple syrup)**
- **Fat: 12g**
- **Sodium: 350mg (varies with soy sauce content)**
- **Potassium: 500mg**
- **Phosphorus: 150mg**

3. Air Fryer Sweet Potato and Black Bean Burritos

Ingredients:

- 2 medium sweet potatoes, peeled and diced
- 1 can (15 oz) black beans, rinsed and drained
- 1 small red onion, finely chopped
- 1 small red bell pepper, diced
- 1 clove garlic, minced
- 1 teaspoon ground cumin
- 1 teaspoon chili powder
- 1/2 teaspoon smoked paprika
- 1/4 teaspoon ground black pepper
- 1/4 teaspoon salt (optional, check with your dietitian)
- 1 tablespoon olive oil
- 1/4 cup fresh cilantro, chopped (optional)
- 4 large whole wheat tortillas
- 1/2 cup shredded low-fat cheese (optional, check with your dietitian)
- Olive oil spray

For Serving:

- Salsa (optional, check with your dietitian)
- Avocado slices (optional, check with your dietitian)

- Lime wedges

Instructions:

1. Set your air fryer's temperature for three to five minutes at 375°F (190°C).
2. Combine the diced sweet potatoes, black pepper, smoked paprika, chili powder, ground cumin, and olive oil in a big bowl. Toss until the potatoes are uniformly coated.
3. To keep the air fryer basket from sticking, lightly mist it with olive oil spray.
4. Arrange the seasoned sweet potatoes in a single layer within the air fryer basket. Sweet potatoes should be cooked for 15 to 20 minutes, shaking the basket halfway through, or until they are soft and beginning to crisp up.
5. In a sizable mixing basin, mix the black beans, minced garlic, diced red bell pepper, chopped onion, and chopped cilantro (if using) while the sweet potatoes are cooking.
6. Add the cooked sweet potatoes to the black bean mixture and gently toss to incorporate.
7. To make the tortillas more malleable, briefly reheat them in the microwave or on the stovetop.
8. Fill the middle of each tortilla with some of the sweet potato and black bean mixture. If using, top with shredded cheese.

9. To create a burrito, carefully roll up each tortilla, tucking in the edges as you roll.

10. Reapply a little coat of olive oil spray to the air fryer basket. Put the burritos into the air fryer basket, seam side down. The number of batches you need to cook them in will depend on how big your air fryer is.

11. Gently mist the burritos' tops with olive oil spray.

12. Bake the burritos in the air fryer for 5 to 7 minutes, or until the tortillas are crispy and golden brown, at 375°F (190°C).

13. Using tongs, carefully take the burritos out of the air fryer.

14. Allow them to cool somewhat before serving, if you'd like, with avocado slices, salsa, and lime wedges.

Nutritional Information (per burrito, based on 4 burritos):

- **Calories: 350**
- **Protein: 10g**
- **Carbohydrates: 60g**
- **Dietary Fiber: 12g**
- **Sugars: 7g**
- **Fat: 9g**

- **Sodium: 400mg (varies with salt and cheese content)**
- **Potassium: 700mg**
- **Phosphorus: 150mg**

4. *Air Fryer Quinoa and Veggie-Stuffed Tomatoes*

Ingredients:

- 4 large tomatoes
- 1 cup cooked quinoa
- 1/2 cup canned black beans, rinsed and drained
- 1 small zucchini, finely diced
- 1 small red bell pepper, finely diced
- 1 small onion, finely chopped
- 1 clove garlic, minced
- 1 tablespoon olive oil
- 1 teaspoon ground cumin
- 1/2 teaspoon chili powder
- 1/4 teaspoon ground black pepper
- 1/4 teaspoon salt (optional, check with your dietitian)
- 1/4 cup grated Parmesan cheese (optional, check with your dietitian)
- Fresh parsley or cilantro for garnish (optional)

Instructions:

1. Set your air fryer's temperature for three to five minutes at 375°F (190°C).

2. Slice off the tops of the tomatoes and use a spoon to remove the insides, taking cautious not to pierce the outer walls. Remove the scooped-out meat and set aside the tomato tops.

3. Heat the olive oil in a big pan over medium heat. Add the red bell pepper, chopped onion, minced garlic, and cubed zucchini. Sauté for approximately five minutes, or until the veggies are tender.

4. Add the black beans, cooked quinoa, chili powder, ground cumin, black pepper, and salt (if needed). Cook for a further two to three minutes, or until well heated. Take off the heat.

5. Stuff the quinoa and vegetable mixture into each hollowed-out tomato, lightly pushing to compact the filling.

6. Top each filled tomato, if using, with a little pinch of grated Parmesan cheese.

7. To keep the air fryer basket from sticking, lightly mist it with olive oil spray.

8. Arrange the filled tomatoes in a single layer within the air fryer basket. The number of batches you need to cook them in will depend on how big your air fryer is.

9. Cook the stuffed tomatoes for 10 to 12 minutes, or until the tomatoes are soft and the filling is well

cooked, at 375°F (190°C). If cheese is being used, it must be bubbling and melted.

10. Using tongs, carefully take the filled tomatoes out of the air fryer.

11. Before serving, let them cool somewhat.

12. If preferred, garnish with fresh cilantro or parsley.

Nutritional Information (per stuffed tomato, based on 4 servings):

- **Calories: 200**
- **Protein: 7g**
- **Carbohydrates: 28g**
- **Dietary Fiber: 6g**
- **Sugars: 8g**
- **Fat: 7g**
- **Sodium: 250mg (varies with salt and cheese content)**
- **Potassium: 600mg**
- **Phosphorus: 100mg**

5. Air Fryer Eggplant and Chickpea Curry

Ingredients:

- 1 large eggplant, diced into 1-inch cubes
- 1 can (15 oz) chickpeas, rinsed and drained
- 1 small onion, finely chopped
- 1 small red bell pepper, diced
- 1 clove garlic, minced
- 1 tablespoon olive oil
- 1 can (14.5 oz) diced tomatoes (no salt added)
- 1/2 cup coconut milk (light or regular)
- 1 tablespoon curry powder
- 1 teaspoon ground cumin
- 1 teaspoon ground coriander
- 1/2 teaspoon ground turmeric
- 1/4 teaspoon ground black pepper
- 1/4 teaspoon salt (optional, check with your dietitian)
- Fresh cilantro for garnish (optional)
- Cooked brown rice or quinoa for serving

Instructions:

1. Set your air fryer's temperature for three to five minutes at 375°F (190°C).
2. Evenly cover the diced eggplant in a big bowl with 1/2 tablespoon olive oil, ground black pepper, and salt (if using).
3. To keep the air fryer basket from sticking, lightly mist it with olive oil spray.
4. Arrange the seasoned eggplant in a single layer within the air fryer basket. Cook, shaking the basket

halfway through, until the eggplant is soft and beginning to crisp up, 15 to 20 minutes.

5. Heat the remaining 1/2 tablespoon of olive oil in a big pan over medium heat while the eggplant is frying. Add the minced garlic, chopped onion, and diced red bell pepper. Sauté for approximately five minutes, or until the veggies are tender.

6. Add the ground turmeric, ground coriander, ground cumin, and curry powder. Cook until the spices become aromatic, one to two minutes.

7. Fill the skillet with the chopped tomatoes and coconut milk, together with their juice. Mix everything together.

8. Fill the pan with the drained and washed chickpeas. Mix everything together.

9. Transfer the cooked eggplant to the skillet. Gently mix all the ingredients together.

10. Simmer the curry for ten to fifteen minutes to let the spices combine and the sauce gradually thicken.

11. Serve the eggplant and chickpeas curry with cooked quinoa or brown rice.

12. If preferred, garnish with fresh cilantro.

Nutritional Information (per serving, based on 4 servings, without rice or quinoa):

- **Calories: 200**
- **Protein: 5g**
- **Carbohydrates: 27g**

- **Dietary Fiber: 8g**
- **Sugars: 10g**
- **Fat: 9g**
- **Sodium: 200mg (varies with salt content)**
- **Potassium: 600mg**
- **Phosphorus: 100mg**

6. Air Fryer Barley and Vegetable Casserole

Ingredients:

- 1 cup pearl barley
- 2 cups low-sodium vegetable broth
- 1/2 cup diced carrots
- 1/2 cup diced bell peppers (any color)
- 1/2 cup diced zucchini
- 1/2 cup diced onions
- 1/2 cup chopped broccoli florets
- 2 cloves garlic, minced
- 1 tsp dried thyme
- 1 tsp dried oregano
- 1/2 tsp ground black pepper
- 1/4 tsp salt
- 1 tbsp olive oil
- 1/4 cup grated Parmesan cheese (optional)

- Non-stick spray

Instructions:

1. Follow the directions on the package to cook the pearl barley in the low-sodium vegetable broth. Usually, this takes between 25 and 30 minutes. After cooking, place it aside.

2. Set the air fryer's temperature for three minutes to 350°F/175°C.

3. Add the chopped broccoli florets, bell peppers, zucchini, onions, and diced carrots to a large mixing bowl.

4. Combine the vegetable combination with the minced garlic, olive oil, salt, crushed black pepper, dried thyme, and dried oregano. Toss until the oil and spices are distributed equally over the veggies.

5. Use a little amount of nonstick spray to coat a casserole dish or oven-safe baking dish that fits within the air fryer basket.

6. Evenly distribute the cooked barley across the casserole dish.

7. Evenly spoon the seasoned vegetable mixture over the barley on top of it.

8. To keep the veggies from drying out, cover the casserole dish with aluminum foil.

9. Insert the casserole dish into the basket of the air fryer.

10. Air fried the veggies for 20 to 25 minutes, or until they are soft, at 350°F/175°C.

11. Take off the foil and sprinkle the Parmesan cheese on top of the casserole, if using. Put the dish back in the air fryer and let it cook for a further three to five minutes, or until the cheese is bubbling and melted.

12. Before serving, carefully take the casserole dish out of the air fryer and allow it to cool for a few minutes.

Nutritional Information (per serving, based on 6 servings without Parmesan cheese):

- **Calories: 200**
- **Protein: 5g**
- **Carbohydrates: 38g**
- **Dietary Fiber: 7g**
- **Sugars: 4g**
- **Total Fat: 4g**
- **Saturated Fat: 0.5g**
- **Sodium: 250mg**
- **Potassium: 300mg**

7. Crispy Air Fryer Cauliflower and Chickpea Tacos

Ingredients:

- 1 small head cauliflower, cut into small florets
- 1 can (15 oz) chickpeas, drained and rinsed
- 2 tbsp olive oil
- 1 tsp ground cumin
- 1 tsp smoked paprika
- 1/2 tsp garlic powder
- 1/2 tsp onion powder
- 1/4 tsp black pepper
- 1/4 tsp salt
- 8 small whole-grain tortillas
- 1/2 cup shredded lettuce
- 1/2 cup diced tomatoes
- 1/4 cup diced red onion
- 1/4 cup chopped fresh cilantro
- Lime wedges for serving
- Non-stick spray

Instructions:

1. For three minutes, preheat the air fryer to 375°F (190°C).
2. Put the chickpeas and cauliflower florets in a large mixing dish.
3. Give the chickpeas and cauliflower a drizzle of olive oil. Incorporate the smoked paprika, ground cumin, onion and garlic powders, black pepper, and

salt. Toss to cover the chickpeas and cauliflower in a uniform layer of oil and spices.

4. Lightly mist the nonstick spray on the air fryer basket.

5. Arrange the chickpeas and seasoned cauliflower in a single layer within the air fryer basket.

6. Air fry the cauliflower for 15 to 20 minutes at 375°F (190°C), shaking the basket halfway through, or until it's crispy and soft and the chickpeas are crunchy and golden.

7. Chop the fresh cilantro, cube the tomatoes and red onion, and shred the lettuce for the taco toppings while the cauliflower and chickpeas are cooking.

8. Heat the whole-grain tortillas in the air fryer for one to two minutes, or until they are soft and malleable, after the cauliflower and chickpeas are done.

9. Top each tortilla with some of the cooked cauliflower and chickpeas to make the tacos.

10. Add chopped cilantro, diced tomatoes, diced red onion, and shredded lettuce on top.

11. Present the tacos with lime wedges on the side for squeezing.

12. Savor right away.

Nutritional Information (per taco, based on 8 tacos):

- Calories: 180
- Protein: 6g
- Carbohydrates: 28g
- Dietary Fiber: 6g
- Sugars: 3g
- Total Fat: 6g
- Saturated Fat: 1g
- Sodium: 250mg
- Potassium: 400mg

8. Air Fryer Stuffed Bell Peppers

Ingredients:

- 4 large bell peppers (any color)
- 1 cup cooked quinoa
- 1 can (15 oz) black beans, drained and rinsed
- 1/2 cup corn kernels (fresh, canned, or frozen)
- 1 small onion, diced
- 1/2 cup diced tomatoes
- 1/2 cup shredded low-fat cheese (optional)
- 1 tsp ground cumin
- 1 tsp chili powder
- 1/2 tsp garlic powder
- 1/2 tsp onion powder
- 1/4 tsp black pepper
- 1/4 tsp salt
- 1 tbsp olive oil

- Fresh cilantro for garnish (optional)
- Lime wedges for serving
- Non-stick spray

Instructions:

1. For three minutes, preheat the air fryer to 360°F (180°C).

2. Cut off the bell peppers' tops to extract the seeds and membranes. Grease the insides of the peppers with a small amount of nonstick spray.

3. Combine the cooked quinoa, black beans, corn kernels, chopped onion, diced tomatoes, ground cumin, onion, garlic, chili powder, black pepper, olive oil, and salt in a big bowl. Toss to blend thoroughly.

4. Gently push down to cram the filling into each bell pepper after stuffing it with the quinoa and veggie mixture.

5. Top each stuffed pepper with a little quantity of cheese, if using.

6. Ensure that the stuffed bell peppers are arranged upright and apart from one another in the air fryer basket.

7. Air fry for 15 to 20 minutes, or until the peppers are soft and the filling is well cooked, at 360°F (180°C). Cook the cheese, if using, until it's bubbling and melted.

8. Before serving, carefully take the stuffed peppers out of the air fryer and allow them to cool for a few minutes.

9. Serve with lime wedges on the side and garnish with fresh cilantro.

Nutritional Information (per stuffed pepper, based on 4 servings without cheese):

- **Calories: 250**
- **Protein: 8g**
- **Carbohydrates: 45g**
- **Dietary Fiber: 10g**
- **Sugars: 8g**
- **Total Fat: 6g**
- **Saturated Fat: 1g**
- **Sodium: 320mg**
- **Potassium: 600mg**

9. Air Fryer Broccoli and Tofu Stir-Fry

Ingredients:

- 1 block (14 oz) firm tofu, drained and pressed
- 2 cups broccoli florets
- 1 red bell pepper, sliced

- 1 small onion, sliced
- 2 cloves garlic, minced
- 2 tbsp low-sodium soy sauce
- 1 tbsp olive oil
- 1 tbsp cornstarch
- 1 tsp sesame oil (optional)
- 1/2 tsp ground ginger
- 1/4 tsp black pepper
- 1/4 tsp red pepper flakes (optional)
- Cooked brown rice or quinoa for serving
- Fresh sesame seeds and green onions for garnish (optional)
- Non-stick spray

Instructions:

1. For three minutes, preheat the air fryer to 375°F (190°C).
2. Create 1-inch cubes out of the pressed tofu.
3. Make sure the tofu cubes are equally covered by tossing them with cornstarch in a big dish.
4. Lightly mist the nonstick spray on the air fryer basket. Arrange the tofu cubes in a single layer within the basket.
5. Shake the basket halfway through the tofu's air-frying process at 375°F (190°C) for 12 to 15 minutes, or until the tofu turns golden and crisp.
6. Prepare the veggies while the tofu is cooking. Broccoli florets, sliced red bell pepper, sliced onion,

and minced garlic should all be combined in a large mixing dish.

7. Combine the olive oil, sesame oil (if using), ground ginger, black pepper, red pepper flakes, and low-sodium soy sauce in a small dish.

8. Drizzle the veggies with the soy sauce mixture and toss to cover well.

9. Take the tofu out of the air fryer and place it aside once it's finished.

10. Fill the air fryer basket with the seasoned veggies. Vegetables should be air-fried for 10 to 12 minutes at 375°F (190°C), shaking the basket halfway through, until they are crisp but still soft.

11. Toss the cooked tofu into the air fryer basket with the veggies, and air fry for a further two to three minutes to heat through and blend flavors.

12. Take the stir-fry out of the air fryer and serve it over quinoa or brown rice that has been cooked.

13. If preferred, garnish with chopped green onions and fresh sesame seeds. Warm up and savor.

Nutritional Information (per serving, based on 4 servings without rice or quinoa):

- **Calories: 200**
- **Protein: 12g**
- **Carbohydrates: 15g**
- **Dietary Fiber: 4g**
- **Sugars: 4g**

- **Total Fat: 10g**
- **Saturated Fat: 1.5g**
- **Sodium: 350mg**
- **Potassium: 500mg**

10. Air Fryer Butternut Squash and Lentil Salad

Ingredients:

- 2 cups butternut squash, peeled and diced
- 1 can (15 oz) lentils, drained and rinsed
- 1 small red onion, diced
- 1/2 cup cherry tomatoes, halved
- 1/4 cup chopped fresh parsley
- 2 tbsp olive oil
- 1 tbsp balsamic vinegar
- 1 tsp ground cumin
- 1/2 tsp paprika
- 1/2 tsp garlic powder
- 1/4 tsp black pepper
- 1/4 tsp salt
- 2 cups mixed greens (spinach, arugula, or kale)
- Non-stick spray

Instructions:

1. For three minutes, preheat the air fryer to 375°F (190°C).

2. Combine the diced butternut squash, 1 tablespoon olive oil, paprika, ground cumin, garlic powder, black pepper, and salt in a large bowl and toss until the squash is well coated.

3. Lightly mist the nonstick spray on the air fryer basket. Arrange the seasoned butternut squash in a single layer into the basket.

4. Until the squash is soft and golden brown, air fry it at 375°F (190°C) for 15 to 20 minutes, shaking the basket halfway through.

5. Make the salad while the squash is cooking. Drained lentils, chopped parsley, sliced red onion, and half-cut cherry tomatoes should all be combined in a big mixing basin.

6. To prepare the dressing, combine the remaining 1 tablespoon olive oil and balsamic vinegar in a small dish.

7. Allow the butternut squash to cool slightly after cooking it before combining it with the salad.

8. Include the butternut squash that has been air-fried in the lentil mixture and stir thoroughly.

9. Pour the salad dressing over it and gently mix to cover all the ingredients.

10. Put the combined greens onto many plates or a large serving dish.

11. Spread the lentil and butternut squash mixture over the mixed greens.

12. Present right away and savor.

Nutritional Information (per serving, based on 4 servings):

- **Calories: 220**
- **Protein: 7g**
- **Carbohydrates: 30g**
- **Dietary Fiber: 10g**
- **Sugars: 6g**
- **Total Fat: 8g**
- **Saturated Fat: 1g**
- **Sodium: 300mg**
- **Potassium: 600mg**

11. Air Fryer Falafel with Whole Grain Pita

Ingredients:

- 1 can (15 oz) chickpeas, drained and rinsed
- 1/4 cup chopped onion
- 2 cloves garlic, minced
- 1/4 cup chopped fresh parsley
- 1/4 cup chopped fresh cilantro
- 2 tbsp whole wheat flour
- 1 tsp ground cumin

- 1 tsp ground coriander
- 1/2 tsp baking powder
- 1/2 tsp paprika
- 1/4 tsp salt
- 1/4 tsp black pepper
- 1 tbsp olive oil
- Non-stick spray
- Whole grain pita bread
- **Toppings:** diced tomatoes, sliced cucumbers, shredded lettuce, tahini sauce, lemon wedges

Instructions:

1. Preheat the air fryer to 375°F (190°C) for 3 minutes.
2. In a food processor, combine the chickpeas, chopped onion, minced garlic, parsley, cilantro, whole wheat flour, ground cumin, ground coriander, baking powder, paprika, salt, and black pepper.
3. Pulse the mixture until it is well combined but still slightly chunky. Be careful not to over-process; the mixture should hold together when formed into balls.
4. Transfer the falafel mixture to a bowl. Using your hands, form the mixture into small balls or patties, about 1-2 inches in diameter. You should get about 12 falafel balls.

5. Lightly spray the air fryer basket with non-stick spray. Place the falafel balls in the basket in a single layer, making sure they do not touch each other.

6. Lightly brush the falafel balls with olive oil to help them crisp up.

7. Air fry the falafel at 375°F (190°C) for 12-15 minutes, shaking the basket halfway through, until the falafel are golden brown and crispy.

8. While the falafel is cooking, warm the whole grain pita bread in the air fryer for 1-2 minutes until soft and pliable.

9. Once the falafel are done, remove them from the air fryer and let them cool for a few minutes.

10. To serve, cut the warmed pita bread in half and open to form pockets.

11. Fill each pita half with a few falafel balls and your choice of toppings: diced tomatoes, sliced cucumbers, shredded lettuce, and a drizzle of tahini sauce. Serve with lemon wedges on the side.

12. Enjoy the warmth.

Nutritional Information (per serving, based on 4 servings):

- **Calories: 300**
- **Protein: 10g**
- **Carbohydrates: 45g**
- **Dietary Fiber: 10g**
- **Sugars: 3g**

- **Total Fat: 10g**
- **Saturated Fat: 1.5g**
- **Sodium: 400mg**
- **Potassium: 400mg**

12. Air Fryer Zucchini and Black Bean Enchiladas

Ingredients:

- 2 medium zucchinis, diced
- 1 can (15 oz) black beans, drained and rinsed
- 1/2 cup corn kernels (fresh, canned, or frozen)
- 1 small onion, diced
- 1 clove garlic, minced
- 1 cup enchilada sauce (store-bought or homemade)
- 1 cup shredded low-fat cheese (optional)
- 8 small whole grain tortillas
- 1 tbsp olive oil
- 1 tsp ground cumin
- 1 tsp chili powder
- 1/2 tsp paprika
- 1/4 tsp black pepper
- 1/4 tsp salt
- Fresh cilantro for garnish (optional)
- Non-stick spray

Instructions:

1. For three minutes, preheat the air fryer to 375°F (190°C).
2. Heat the olive oil in a big skillet over medium heat. Add the chopped onion and simmer for 3–4 minutes, or until it turns transparent.
3. Add the minced garlic and stir until fragrant, about 1 more minute.
4. Fill the pan with the diced zucchini, black beans, and corn kernels. Mix everything together.
5. Add salt, black pepper, paprika, chili powder, and powdered cumin to the mixture. Sauté the zucchini for 5 to 7 minutes, or until they are soft.
6. Use a little amount of nonstick spray to coat a baking dish that fits within the air fryer basket.
7. To keep the baking dish from sticking, lightly coat the bottom with enchilada sauce.
8. Arrange the tortillas in a level fashion. Place a little amount of the black bean and zucchini mixture onto each tortilla, then firmly roll each one.
9. Slide the rolled tortillas into the baking dish, seam side down.
10. Evenly distribute the leftover enchilada sauce on top of the rolled tortillas.
11. Top the enchiladas with the low-fat cheese, if using, that has been shredded.

12. Insert the baking dish into the basket of the air fryer.

13. Air fry the enchiladas for 10 to 15 minutes, or until they are well cooked and the cheese is bubbling and melted, at 375°F (190°C).

14. Before serving, carefully take the baking dish out of the air fryer and allow the enchiladas to cool for a few minutes.

15. If preferred, garnish with fresh cilantro.

16. Serve warm and enjoy.

Nutritional Information (per serving, based on 4 servings):

- **Calories: 350**
- **Protein: 14g**
- **Carbohydrates: 45g**
- **Dietary Fiber: 10g**
- **Sugars: 5g**
- **Total Fat: 12g**
- **Saturated Fat: 3g**
- **Sodium: 600mg**
- **Potassium: 700mg**

CHAPTER SIX: CRUNCHY KIDNEY TRANSPLANT AIR FRYER SNACKS AND APPETIZER

Welcome to the Kidney Transplant Air Fryer Diet Cookbook's snack and appetizer section. This assortment includes a selection of delightful, kidney-friendly bites suitable for any time of day. From crispy veggie chips to savory nibbles, these recipes employ the flexible air fryer to create quick, simple, and healthful meals. Enjoy these delectable snacks and appetizers that fulfill appetites while also benefiting your health.

1. Air Fryer Kale Chips

Ingredients:

- 1 bunch kale
- 1 tbsp olive oil

- 1/2 tsp garlic powder
- 1/4 tsp smoked paprika
- 1/4 tsp salt
- 1/4 tsp black pepper

Instructions:

1. For three minutes, preheat the air fryer to 350°F (175°C).
2. Give the kale leaves a thorough wash and drying. Tear the leaves into bite-sized pieces after removing the stiff stems.
3. Make sure the kale pieces are equally coated by tossing them with olive oil in a large mixing dish.
4. Top the kale with a pinch of salt, black pepper, smoky paprika, and garlic powder. To evenly distribute the spices, toss again.
5. Lightly mist the nonstick spray on the air fryer basket.
6. Arrange the seasoned kale leaves in a single layer within the air fryer basket. It could be necessary to work in batches in order to prevent overcrowding.
7. To achieve consistent frying, air fry for five to seven minutes at 350°F (175°C), shaking the basket halfway through. To avoid scorching the kale, pay great attention to it.
8. Carefully take the crispy, slightly browned kale chips out of the air fryer.

9. Before serving, let the kale chips cool for a few minutes. When they cool, they will keep getting crispier.

10. Consume right away or keep at room temperature for up to two days in an airtight container.

Nutritional Information (per serving, based on 4 servings):

- **Calories: 60**
- **Protein: 2g**
- **Carbohydrates: 6g**
- **Dietary Fiber: 2g**
- **Sugars: 0g**
- **Total Fat: 3.5g**
- **Saturated Fat: 0.5g**
- **Sodium: 150mg**
- **Potassium: 300mg**

2. Air Fryer Chickpeas

Ingredients:

- 1 can (15 oz) chickpeas, drained and rinsed
- 1 tbsp olive oil
- 1/2 tsp garlic powder
- 1/2 tsp smoked paprika

- 1/4 tsp ground cumin
- 1/4 tsp black pepper
- 1/4 tsp salt

Instructions:

1. For three minutes, preheat the air fryer to 375°F (190°C).

2. Use paper towels to pat the washed and drained chickpeas dry. Squeezing out as much moisture as you can will make them crispier.

3. Make sure the chickpeas are uniformly covered by tossing them with olive oil in a large mixing dish.

4. Drizzle the chickpeas with the smoked paprika, ground cumin, black pepper, garlic powder, and salt. In order to spread the spices equally, toss again.

5. Lightly mist the nonstick spray on the air fryer basket.

6. Spread out the seasoned chickpeas in a single layer within the air fryer basket.

7. To achieve consistent cooking, air fry for 12 to 15 minutes at 375°F (190°C), shaking the basket halfway through. Observe the chickpeas closely to avoid scorching them.

8. Carefully take the chickpeas out of the air fryer after they are crispy and golden brown.

9. Before serving, allow the chickpeas to cool for a few minutes. When they cool, they will keep getting crispier.

10. Consume right away or keep at room temperature for up to two days in an airtight container.

Nutritional Information (per serving, based on 4 servings):

- **Calories: 120**
- **Protein: 5g**
- **Carbohydrates: 18g**
- **Dietary Fiber: 5g**
- **Sugars: 1g**
- **Total Fat: 4g**
- **Saturated Fat: 0.5g**
- **Sodium: 200mg**
- **Potassium: 200mg**

3. Air Fryer Sweet Potato Fries

Ingredients:

- 2 medium sweet potatoes
- 1 tbsp olive oil
- 1/2 tsp garlic powder
- 1/2 tsp paprika

- 1/4 tsp black pepper
- 1/4 tsp salt
- Non-stick spray

Instructions:

1. For three minutes, preheat the air fryer to 375°F (190°C).
2. After peeling, cut the sweet potatoes into fries that are around 1/4 inch thick and of uniform size.
3. Make sure the sweet potato fries are equally coated by tossing them with olive oil in a large mixing dish.
4. Dust the fries with salt, black pepper, paprika, and garlic powder. In order to spread the spices equally, toss again.
5. Lightly mist the nonstick spray on the air fryer basket.
6. Spread out the seasoned sweet potato fries in a single layer within the air fryer basket. To prevent crowding, you might need to cook them in batches, depending on how big your air fryer is.
7. To achieve consistent frying, air fry for 15 to 20 minutes at 375°F (190°C), shaking the basket halfway through. Since air fryers differ in terms of doneness, make any necessary adjustments to the cooking time.
8. Carefully take the sweet potato fries out of the air fryer after they are golden brown and crispy.

9. Before serving, let the fries cool for a few minutes. When they cool, they will keep getting crispier.

10. Present right away and savor.

Nutritional Information (per serving, based on 4 servings):

- **Calories: 140**
- **Protein: 2g**
- **Carbohydrates: 26g**
- **Dietary Fiber: 4g**
- **Sugars: 5g**
- **Total Fat: 4g**
- **Saturated Fat: 0.5g**
- **Sodium: 200mg**
- **Potassium: 400mg**

4. Air Fryer Zucchini Chips

Ingredients:

- 2 medium zucchinis
- 1 tbsp olive oil
- 1/2 cup whole wheat breadcrumbs
- 1/4 cup grated Parmesan cheese (optional)
- 1/2 tsp garlic powder
- 1/2 tsp onion powder

- 1/4 tsp paprika
- 1/4 tsp black pepper
- 1/4 tsp salt
- Non-stick spray

Instructions:

1. For three minutes, preheat the air fryer to 375°F (190°C).
2. Rinse the zucchini and cut thin rounds out of them, about 1/8 inch thick.
3. Make sure the zucchini slices are equally coated by tossing them with olive oil in a large mixing dish.
4. Transfer the whole wheat breadcrumbs, grated Parmesan cheese (if desired), paprika, onion, garlic, black pepper, and salt to a different bowl. Blend well.
5. To make sure the crumbs adhere to all sides, dip each zucchini slice into the breadcrumb mixture and gently press.
6. Lightly mist the nonstick spray on the air fryer basket.
7. Fill the air fryer basket with the coated zucchini slices arranged in a single layer. Cooking them in batches might be necessary to prevent crowding.
8. Air fry the zucchini chips for 8 to 10 minutes at 375°F (190°C), shaking the basket halfway through, or until they are crispy and golden brown.

9. Before serving, carefully take the zucchini chips out of the air fryer and allow them to cool for a few minutes. When they cool, they will keep getting crispier.

10. Present right away and savor.

Nutritional Information (per serving, based on 4 servings without Parmesan cheese):

- **Calories: 90**
- **Protein: 3g**
- **Carbohydrates: 12g**
- **Dietary Fiber: 2g**
- **Sugars: 3g**
- **Total Fat: 4g**
- **Saturated Fat: 0.5g**
- **Sodium: 200mg**
- **Potassium: 350mg**

5. Air Fryer Stuffed Mini Peppers

Ingredients:

- 12 mini bell peppers
- 1/2 cup cooked quinoa
- 1 can (15 oz) black beans, drained and rinsed
- 1/2 cup corn kernels (fresh, canned, or frozen)
- 1/4 cup diced tomatoes

- 1/4 cup chopped green onions
- 1/4 cup shredded low-fat cheese (optional)
- 1 tsp ground cumin
- 1/2 tsp chili powder
- 1/2 tsp garlic powder
- 1/4 tsp black pepper
- 1/4 tsp salt
- 1 tbsp olive oil
- Fresh cilantro for garnish (optional)
- Non-stick spray

Instructions:

1. Preheat the air fryer to 375°F (190°C) for 3 minutes.
2. Cut the tops off the mini bell peppers and remove the seeds and membranes.
3. In a large mixing bowl, combine the cooked quinoa, black beans, corn kernels, diced tomatoes, and chopped green onions.
4. Add the ground cumin, chili powder, garlic powder, black pepper, and salt to the mixture. Stir to combine.
5. If using, add the shredded low-fat cheese to the mixture and stir until evenly distributed.
6. Stuff each mini bell pepper with the quinoa and vegetable mixture, pressing down lightly to pack the filling.

7. Lightly spray the air fryer basket with non-stick spray.

8. Arrange the stuffed mini peppers in the air fryer basket in a single layer.

9. Lightly brush the tops of the stuffed peppers with olive oil to help them crisp up.

10. Air fry at 375°F (190°C) for 10-12 minutes, or until the peppers are tender and the filling is heated through.

11. Carefully remove the stuffed mini peppers from the air fryer and let them cool for a few minutes before serving.

12. Garnish with fresh cilantro if desired.

13. Serve warm and enjoy.

Nutritional Information (per serving, based on 4 servings):

- **Calories: 180**
- **Protein: 6g**
- **Carbohydrates: 28g**
- **Dietary Fiber: 7g**
- **Sugars: 6g**
- **Total Fat: 6g**
- **Saturated Fat: 1g**
- **Sodium: 300mg**
- **Potassium: 500mg**

6. Air Fryer Cauliflower Bites

Ingredients:

- 1 medium head of cauliflower, cut into bite-sized florets
- 1/2 cup whole wheat breadcrumbs
- 1/4 cup grated Parmesan cheese (optional)
- 1 tsp garlic powder
- 1/2 tsp paprika
- 1/2 tsp onion powder
- 1/4 tsp black pepper
- 1/4 tsp salt
- 2 large eggs
- 1 tbsp olive oil
- Non-stick spray

Instructions:

1. Preheat the air fryer to 375°F (190°C) for 3 minutes.
2. In a large mixing bowl, combine the whole wheat breadcrumbs, grated Parmesan cheese (if using), garlic powder, paprika, onion powder, black pepper, and salt. Mix well.
3. In another bowl, beat the eggs.
4. Dip each cauliflower floret into the beaten eggs, ensuring it is fully coated.

5. Transfer the egg-coated cauliflower to the breadcrumb mixture and toss to coat evenly. Press lightly to ensure the breadcrumbs stick to the florets.

6. Lightly spray the air fryer basket with non-stick spray.

7. Place the coated cauliflower florets in the air fryer basket in a single layer. You may need to cook them in batches to avoid overcrowding.

8. Lightly brush or spray the tops of the cauliflower florets with olive oil to help them crisp up.

9. Air fry at 375°F (190°C) for 12-15 minutes, shaking the basket halfway through, until the cauliflower bites are golden brown and crispy.

10. Carefully remove the cauliflower bites from the air fryer and let them cool for a few minutes before serving.

11. Serve warm with your favorite dipping sauce.

Nutritional Information (per serving, based on 4 servings):

- **Calories: 140**
- **Protein: 7g**
- **Carbohydrates: 16g**
- **Dietary Fiber: 4g**
- **Sugars: 2g**
- **Total Fat: 6g**
- **Saturated Fat: 1.5g**

- Sodium: 280mg
- Potassium: 450mg

7. Air Fryer Apple Chips

Ingredients:

- 2 medium apples (any variety)
- 1/2 tsp ground cinnamon
- 1/4 tsp ground nutmeg (optional)
- Non-stick spray

Instructions:

1. Preheat the air fryer to 300°F (150°C) for 3 minutes.
2. Wash and core the apples. Using a mandoline or a sharp knife, thinly slice the apples into rounds about 1/8 inch thick.
3. In a large mixing bowl, toss the apple slices with ground cinnamon and ground nutmeg (if using), ensuring they are evenly coated.
4. Lightly spray the air fryer basket with non-stick spray.
5. Place the apple slices in the air fryer basket in a single layer, ensuring they do not overlap. You may need to cook them in batches to avoid overcrowding.

6. Air fry at 300°F (150°C) for 15-20 minutes, flipping the apple slices halfway through the cooking time. Keep a close eye on them to prevent burning.

7. Once the apple slices are crispy and lightly browned, carefully remove them from the air fryer.

8. Let the apple chips cool for a few minutes before serving. They will continue to crisp up as they cool.

9. Enjoy immediately or store in an airtight container at room temperature for up to 3 days.

Nutritional Information (per serving, based on 4 servings):

- **Calories: 60**
- **Protein: 0.5g**
- **Carbohydrates: 16g**
- **Dietary Fiber: 3g**
- **Sugars: 12g**
- **Total Fat: 0g**
- **Saturated Fat: 0g**
- **Sodium: 0mg**
- **Potassium: 120mg**

8. Air Fryer Avocado Fries

Ingredients:

- 2 ripe avocados
- 1/2 cup whole wheat breadcrumbs
- 1/4 cup grated Parmesan cheese (optional)
- 1/2 tsp garlic powder
- 1/2 tsp paprika
- 1/4 tsp black pepper
- 1/4 tsp salt
- 2 large eggs
- Non-stick spray

Instructions:

1. Preheat the air fryer to 375°F (190°C) for 3 minutes.
2. Cut the avocados in half, remove the pits, and slice each half into wedges.
3. In a large mixing bowl, combine the whole wheat breadcrumbs, grated Parmesan cheese (if using), garlic powder, paprika, black pepper, and salt. Mix well.
4. In another bowl, beat the eggs.
5. Dip each avocado wedge into the beaten eggs, ensuring it is fully coated.
6. Transfer the egg-coated avocado wedge to the breadcrumb mixture and toss to coat evenly. Press lightly to ensure the breadcrumbs stick to the wedges.
7. Lightly spray the air fryer basket with non-stick spray.

8. Place the coated avocado wedges in the air fryer basket in a single layer. You may need to cook them in batches to avoid overcrowding.

9. Lightly spray the tops of the avocado wedges with non-stick spray to help them crisp up.

10. Air fry at 375°F (190°C) for 8-10 minutes, flipping halfway through, until the avocado fries are golden brown and crispy.

11. Carefully remove the avocado fries from the air fryer and let them cool for a few minutes before serving.

12. Serve warm with your favorite dipping sauce.

Nutritional Information (per serving, based on 4 servings without Parmesan cheese):

- **Calories: 160**
- **Protein: 4g**
- **Carbohydrates: 13g**
- **Dietary Fiber: 7g**
- **Sugars: 1g**
- **Total Fat: 12g**
- **Saturated Fat: 2g**
- **Sodium: 200mg**
- **Potassium: 450mg**

9. Air Fryer Lentil Meatballs

Ingredients:

- 1 cup cooked green or brown lentils
- 1/2 cup rolled oats
- 1/4 cup grated Parmesan cheese (optional)
- 1/4 cup finely chopped onion
- 2 cloves garlic, minced
- 1/4 cup chopped fresh parsley
- 1 large egg
- 1 tsp dried oregano
- 1 tsp dried basil
- 1/2 tsp ground cumin
- 1/2 tsp paprika
- 1/4 tsp black pepper
- 1/4 tsp salt
- Non-stick spray

Instructions:

1. Preheat the air fryer to 375°F (190°C) for 3 minutes.
2. In a food processor, combine the cooked lentils and rolled oats. Pulse until the mixture is well combined but still has some texture.
3. Transfer the lentil mixture to a large mixing bowl. Add the grated Parmesan cheese (if using), chopped onion, minced garlic, chopped parsley, egg, dried oregano, dried basil, ground cumin,

paprika, black pepper, and salt. Mix well until all ingredients are fully incorporated.

4. Using your hands, form the mixture into small balls, about 1-2 inches in diameter. You should get about 12-15 meatballs.

5. Lightly spray the air fryer basket with non-stick spray.

6. Place the lentil meatballs in the air fryer basket in a single layer, making sure they do not touch each other.

7. Air fry at 375°F (190°C) for 10-12 minutes, shaking the basket halfway through, until the meatballs are golden brown and crispy.

8. Carefully remove the meatballs from the air fryer and let them cool for a few minutes before serving.

9. Serve warm with your favorite marinara sauce or as part of a meal.

Nutritional Information (per serving, based on 4 servings without Parmesan cheese):

- **Calories: 140**
- **Protein: 8g**
- **Carbohydrates: 21g**
- **Dietary Fiber: 7g**
- **Sugars: 1g**
- **Total Fat: 3g**
- **Saturated Fat: 0.5g**
- **Sodium: 180mg**

- **Potassium: 350mg**

10. Air Fryer Broccoli Tots

Ingredients:

- 2 cups fresh broccoli florets
- 1 large egg
- 1/2 cup shredded cheddar cheese (optional)
- 1/4 cup grated Parmesan cheese (optional)
- 1/2 cup whole wheat breadcrumbs
- 1/4 cup finely chopped onion
- 1 clove garlic, minced
- 1/2 tsp garlic powder
- 1/2 tsp onion powder
- 1/4 tsp black pepper
- 1/4 tsp salt
- Non-stick spray

Instructions:

1. Preheat the air fryer to 375°F (190°C) for 3 minutes.
2. Steam or blanch the broccoli florets until they are tender, then drain and let them cool.

3. Finely chop the cooled broccoli florets, or pulse them in a food processor until they are in small pieces.

4. In a large mixing bowl, combine the chopped broccoli, egg, shredded cheddar cheese (if using), grated Parmesan cheese (if using), whole wheat breadcrumbs, finely chopped onion, minced garlic, garlic powder, onion powder, black pepper, and salt. Mix well until all ingredients are fully incorporated.

5. Using your hands, form the mixture into small tot shapes, about 1-2 inches in size. You should get about 20-24 tots.

6. Lightly spray the air fryer basket with non-stick spray.

7. Place the broccoli tots in the air fryer basket in a single layer, making sure they do not touch each other.

8. Air fry at 375°F (190°C) for 10-12 minutes, shaking the basket halfway through, until the tots are golden brown and crispy.

9. Carefully remove the broccoli tots from the air fryer and let them cool for a few minutes before serving.

10. Serve warm with your favorite dipping sauce.

Nutritional Information (per serving, based on 4 servings without cheese):

- Calories: 90

- Protein: 4g
- Carbohydrates: 13g
- Dietary Fiber: 3g
- Sugars: 2g
- Total Fat: 2.5g
- Saturated Fat: 0.5g
- Sodium: 220mg
- Potassium: 250mg

11. Air Fryer Carrot Fries

Ingredients:

- 4 large carrots
- 1 tbsp olive oil
- 1/2 tsp garlic powder
- 1/2 tsp paprika
- 1/4 tsp black pepper
- 1/4 tsp salt
- Non-stick spray

Instructions:

1. For three minutes, preheat the air fryer to 375°F (190°C).
2. After peeling, cut the carrots into sticks that are 3–4 inches long and 1/4 inch thick.

3. Toss the carrot sticks in a big dish of olive oil to make sure they are well coated.

4. Dust the carrots with salt, black pepper, paprika, and garlic powder. In order to spread the spices equally, toss again.

5. Lightly mist the nonstick spray on the air fryer basket.

6. Arrange the seasoned carrot sticks in a single layer into the air fryer basket. Cooking them in batches might be necessary to prevent crowding.

7. Air fry the carrot fries for 12 to 15 minutes at 375°F (190°C), shaking the basket halfway through, or until they are soft and just beginning to crisp.

8. Carefully take the cooked carrot fries out of the air fryer and allow them to cool for a few minutes before serving.

9. Top with your preferred dipping sauce and serve warm.

Nutritional Information (per serving, based on 4 servings):

- **Calories: 80**
- **Protein: 1g**
- **Carbohydrates: 10g**
- **Dietary Fiber: 3g**
- **Sugars: 5g**
- **Total Fat: 4g**
- **Saturated Fat: 0.5g**

- **Sodium: 200mg**
- **Potassium: 300mg**

12. Air Fryer Black Bean Taquitos

Ingredients:

- 1 can (15 oz) black beans, drained and rinsed
- 1/2 cup corn kernels (fresh, canned, or frozen)
- 1/2 cup diced tomatoes
- 1/4 cup diced onions
- 1/4 cup chopped fresh cilantro
- 1 tsp ground cumin
- 1 tsp chili powder
- 1/2 tsp garlic powder
- 1/2 tsp onion powder
- 1/4 tsp black pepper
- 1/4 tsp salt
- 1 cup shredded low-fat cheese (optional)
- 10 small whole grain tortillas
- 1 tbsp olive oil
- Non-stick spray

Instructions:

1. For three minutes, preheat the air fryer to 375°F (190°C).

2. Combine the black beans, corn kernels, chopped cilantro, diced tomatoes, diced onions, ground cumin, chili powder, garlic powder, onion powder, black pepper, and salt in a large mixing bowl. Blend well until all components are dispersed equally.

3. Stir in the shredded cheese, if using, after adding it to the mixture.

4. To make the tortillas more malleable, reheat them in the microwave for 20 to 30 seconds.

5. Spread the black bean mixture in a line down one side of each tortilla, using about 2 teaspoons per tortilla. To create a taquito, firmly roll the tortilla around the filling.

6. Lightly mist the nonstick spray on the air fryer basket.

7. Arrange the taquitos in a single layer in the air fryer basket, seam-side down. Cooking them in batches might be necessary to prevent crowding.

8. To make the taquito tops crisp up, lightly brush them with olive oil.

9. Shake the basket halfway through and air fry the taquitos for 8 to 10 minutes, or until they are crispy and golden brown. The temperature is 375°F (190°C).

10. Before serving, carefully take the taquitos out of the air fryer and allow them to cool for a few minutes.

11. Present warm, accompanied by your preferred salsa or dipping sauce.

Nutritional Information (per serving, based on 10 taquitos):

- Calories: 150
- Protein: 5g
- Carbohydrates: 23g
- Dietary Fiber: 6g
- Sugars: 2g
- Total Fat: 5g
- Saturated Fat: 1g
- Sodium: 250mg
- Potassium: 300mg

CHAPTER SEVEN: YUMMY KIDNEY TRANSPLANT AIR FRYER DESSERT RECIPES

This collection of dessert recipes is specifically designed for individuals who have had a kidney transplant and want to enjoy tasty, kidney-friendly desserts. Our recipes emphasize health-conscious ingredients and simple air fryer procedures, allowing you to indulge without jeopardizing your nutritional goals. From sweet and savory to light and indulgent, each dessert is intended to be both nutritional and filling.

1. Air Fryer Baked Apples

Ingredients:

- 4 medium apples (any variety)

- 1/4 cup rolled oats
- 1/4 cup chopped nuts (walnuts, pecans, or almonds)
- 2 tbsp honey or maple syrup
- 1 tbsp melted butter or coconut oil
- 1 tsp ground cinnamon
- 1/2 tsp ground nutmeg (optional)
- Non-stick spray

Instructions:

1. The air fryer should be preheated for three minutes to 350°F/175°C.
2. Clean the apples and core them, being sure to leave a well for the filling approximately 1/2 inch below the surface. To scoop out the core, use a spoon or a melon baller tool.
3. Combine the ground nutmeg (if using), ground cinnamon, melted butter or coconut oil, chopped nuts, honey or maple syrup, and rolled oats in a small mixing dish. Make sure to thoroughly mix all of the ingredients.
4. Gently press the oat and nut mixture into each apple to ensure that it is fully packed.
5. Use a little nonstick spray to coat the air fryer basket.
6. Pack the filled apples into the air fryer basket in a single layer.

7. Cook the apples for 15-20 minutes, or until they are soft and the filling is browned, at 350°F (175°C) using an air fryer. After halfway done, check the apples and adjust the cooking time if necessary.

8. When ready to serve, carefully take the cooked apples out of the air fryer and allow them to cool.

9. You can choose to serve it warm and add extra honey or maple syrup or a dollop of Greek yogurt on top.

Nutritional Information (per serving, based on 4 servings):

- **Calories: 180**
- **Protein: 2g**
- **Carbohydrates: 30g**
- **Dietary Fiber: 5g**
- **Sugars: 20g**
- **Total Fat: 7g**
- **Saturated Fat: 2g**
- **Sodium: 5mg**
- **Potassium: 220mg**

2. Air Fryer Banana Chips

Ingredients:

- 2 ripe but firm bananas

- 1 tbsp lemon juice
- 1 tbsp water
- Non-stick spray

Instructions:

1. For three minutes, preheat the air fryer to 350°F (175°C).
2. Combine the water and lemon juice in a small bowl.
3. Slice the bananas thinly, about 1/8 inch thick, after peeling them.
4. To avoid browning, gently dip each banana slice into the lemon juice mixture.
5. Lightly mist the nonstick spray on the air fryer basket.
6. Put the banana slices in the air fryer basket in a single layer, being careful not to overlap. Cooking them in batches might be necessary to prevent crowding.
7. Air fry the slices for 8 to 12 minutes at 350°F (175°C), checking and turning them halfway through. Since cooking durations might vary, keep a close check on them to avoid scorching.
8. Carefully take the crispy, golden-brown banana chips out of the air fryer and set them on a wire rack to cool. When they cool, they will keep getting crispier.

9. Savor right away or keep at room temperature for up to two days in an airtight container.

Nutritional Information (per serving, based on 4 servings):

- **Calories: 60**
- **Protein: 0.7g**
- **Carbohydrates: 15g**
- **Dietary Fiber: 2g**
- **Sugars: 8g**
- **Total Fat: 0.2g**
- **Saturated Fat: 0g**
- **Sodium: 0mg**
- **Potassium: 225mg**

3. Air Fryer Oatmeal Cookies

Ingredients:

- 1 cup rolled oats
- 1/2 cup whole wheat flour
- 1/2 cup unsweetened applesauce
- 1/4 cup honey or maple syrup
- 1/4 cup coconut oil, melted
- 1/4 cup raisins or dried cranberries
- 1/4 cup chopped nuts (walnuts or almonds)
- 1 tsp vanilla extract

- 1 tsp ground cinnamon
- 1/2 tsp baking powder
- 1/4 tsp salt

Instructions:

1. For three minutes, preheat the air fryer to 350°F (175°C).
2. Place the rolled oats, whole wheat flour, baking powder, powdered cinnamon, and salt in a large mixing basin. Blend well.
3. In a separate dish, thoroughly mix the melted coconut oil, unsweetened applesauce, honey or maple syrup, and vanilla extract.
4. Add the liquid mixture to the dry mixture and whisk just until blended.
5. Stir in chopped nuts and raisins or dried cranberries.
6. Use parchment paper inside the air fryer basket to stop the cookies from sticking.
7. Using your fingers, gently flatten the tablespoon-sized portions of dough that you have scooped out and placed on the parchment paper. As the cookies cook, they will spread somewhat, so allow some space between them.
8. Air fry the cookies for 8 to 10 minutes, or until they are firm and golden brown, at 350°F (175°C). Midway through the baking time, check the cookies and make any required adjustments.

9. Take the cookies out of the air fryer with caution, and allow them to cool on a wire rack.

10. Consume right away or keep at room temperature for up to a week in an airtight container.

Nutritional Information (per cookie, based on 12 cookies):

- **Calories: 110**
- **Protein: 2g**
- **Carbohydrates: 15g**
- **Dietary Fiber: 2g**
- **Sugars: 7g**
- **Total Fat: 5g**
- **Saturated Fat: 3g**
- **Sodium: 50mg**
- **Potassium: 80mg**

4. Air Fryer Pear Slices with Cinnamon

Ingredients:

- 2 ripe pears
- 1 tsp ground cinnamon
- 1/2 tsp ground nutmeg (optional)

- 1 tsp honey or maple syrup (optional)
- Non-stick spray

Instructions:

1. For three minutes, preheat the air fryer to 350°F (175°C).
2. Give the pears a wash and core. Cut them into wedges that are just 1/4 inch thick.
3. Gently toss the pear slices with ground nutmeg (if using) and cinnamon in a large mixing dish until they are well coated. For added sweetness, feel free to drizzle with honey or maple syrup and toss to coat.
4. Lightly mist the nonstick spray on the air fryer basket.
5. Make sure the pear slices do not overlap when you arrange them in the air fryer basket in a single layer. Cooking them in batches might be necessary to prevent crowding.
6. Air fry the pear slices for 8 to 10 minutes at 350°F (175°C), turning them halfway through, or until they are soft and have a hint of caramel.
7. Before serving, gently take the cooked pear slices out of the air fryer and let them cool for a few minutes.
8. Savor the warm dessert right away.

Nutritional Information (per serving, based on 4 servings):

- Calories: 60
- Protein: 0.5g
- Carbohydrates: 16g
- Dietary Fiber: 3g
- Sugars: 10g
- Total Fat: 0.2g
- Saturated Fat: 0g
- Sodium: 0mg
- Potassium: 120mg

5. Air Fryer Blueberry Quinoa Bars

Ingredients:

- 1 cup cooked quinoa
- 1 cup rolled oats
- 1/4 cup honey or maple syrup
- 1/4 cup almond butter or peanut butter
- 1/4 cup unsweetened applesauce
- 1 tsp vanilla extract
- 1/2 tsp ground cinnamon
- 1/4 tsp salt
- 1 cup fresh or frozen blueberries
- Non-stick spray

Instructions:

1. For three minutes, preheat the air fryer to 350°F (175°C).

2. Put the cooked quinoa, rolled oats, ground cinnamon, honey, maple syrup, almond butter, or peanut butter, unsweetened applesauce, vanilla extract, and salt in a big mixing dish. Blend well until all components are thoroughly blended.

3. Gently incorporate the blueberries into the mixture until they are all mixed together.

4. Lightly apply non-stick spray to a baking dish or pan that is oven safe and fits within the air fryer basket.

5. To ensure that the mixture is packed uniformly, pour the mixture into the baking dish that has been prepared and firmly push down with a spatula.

6. Insert the baking dish into the basket of the air fryer.

7. Air fry the bars for 15 to 20 minutes, or until they are set and have a golden brown top, at 350°F/175°C. Midway during the cooking time, check the bars and make any required adjustments.

8. Before slicing the bars into squares or rectangles, carefully take the baking dish out of the air fryer and allow the bars to cool completely in the dish.

9. Savor right away or keep in the fridge for up to a week or at room temperature for up to three days if stored in an airtight container.

Nutritional Information (per serving, based on 12 bars):

- Calories: 120
- Protein: 3g
- Carbohydrates: 22g
- Dietary Fiber: 3g
- Sugars: 8g
- Total Fat: 3g
- Saturated Fat: 0.5g
- Sodium: 50mg
- Potassium: 100mg

6. Air Fryer Carrot Cake Bites

Ingredients:

- 1 cup grated carrots
- 1/2 cup rolled oats
- 1/4 cup almond flour
- 1/4 cup unsweetened applesauce
- 1/4 cup honey or maple syrup
- 1 large egg
- 1 tsp vanilla extract
- 1 tsp ground cinnamon
- 1/2 tsp ground nutmeg
- 1/2 tsp baking powder

- 1/4 tsp salt
- 1/4 cup chopped walnuts or pecans (optional)
- Non-stick spray

Instructions:

1. For three minutes, preheat the air fryer to 350°F (175°C).
2. Grated carrots, rolled oats, almond flour, unsweetened applesauce, honey or maple syrup, egg, vanilla extract, ground nutmeg, ground cinnamon, baking powder, and salt should all be combined in a big mixing basin. Blend until all components are thoroughly blended.
3. If using, mix in the chopped pecans or walnuts.
4. Lightly mist a small oven-safe dish or silicone muffin cups that fit in your air fryer basket with nonstick cooking spray.
5. Fill each prepared muffin cup or dish about 3/4 of the way to the top with the batter using a spoon.
6. Insert the dish or muffin cups into the air fryer basket.
7. Bake the carrot cake bites for 10 to 12 minutes at 350°F (175°C), or until a toothpick inserted into the middle comes out clean.
8. Take the carrot cake bites out of the air fryer with care, and allow them to cool in the muffin tin or dish for a few minutes before moving them to a wire rack to finish cooling.

9. Savor right away or keep in the fridge for up to a week or at room temperature for up to three days if stored in an airtight container.

Nutritional Information (per serving, based on 12 bites):

- **Calories: 90**
- **Protein: 2g**
- **Carbohydrates: 14g**
- **Dietary Fiber: 2g**
- **Sugars: 7g**
- **Total Fat: 3g**
- **Saturated Fat: 0.5g**
- **Sodium: 70mg**
- **Potassium: 100mg**

7. Air Fryer Sweet Potato Brownies

Ingredients:

- 1 cup mashed sweet potatoes (about 1 medium sweet potato, cooked and mashed)
- 1/2 cup almond flour
- 1/2 cup unsweetened cocoa powder
- 1/4 cup honey or maple syrup
- 1/4 cup almond butter or peanut butter

- 2 large eggs
- 1 tsp vanilla extract
- 1/2 tsp baking powder
- 1/4 tsp salt
- 1/4 cup dark chocolate chips (optional)
- Non-stick spray

Instructions:

1. For three minutes, preheat the air fryer to 325°F (165°C).

2. Put the mashed sweet potatoes, almond flour, unsweetened cocoa powder, eggs, vanilla extract, baking powder, and salt in a big mixing bowl. You may also add honey, maple syrup, almond butter, or peanut butter. Mix until a smooth batter emerges and all ingredients are fully incorporated.

3. If using, fold in the dark chocolate chips.

4. Lightly apply non-stick spray to a baking dish or pan that is oven safe and fits within the air fryer basket.

5. Using a spatula, evenly distribute the batter into the baking dish that has been prepared.

6. Insert the baking dish into the basket of the air fryer.

7. Bake the brownies for 20 to 25 minutes at 325°F (165°C), or until a toothpick inserted into the center comes out clean. Midway through the cooking time,

check the brownies and make any required adjustments.

8. Before slicing the brownies into squares, carefully take the baking dish out of the air fryer and allow the brownies to cool completely in the dish.

9. Savor right away or keep in the fridge for up to a week or at room temperature for up to three days if stored in an airtight container.

Nutritional Information (per serving, based on 12 brownies):

- **Calories: 120**
- **Protein: 3g**
- **Carbohydrates: 15g**
- **Dietary Fiber: 3g**
- **Sugars: 8g**
- **Total Fat: 6g**
- **Saturated Fat: 1.5g**
- **Sodium: 80mg**
- **Potassium: 150mg**

8. Air Fryer Apple Oat Crumble

Ingredients:

For the Filling:

- 4 medium apples (any variety), peeled, cored, and sliced
- 1 tbsp lemon juice
- 1/4 cup honey or maple syrup
- 1 tsp ground cinnamon
- 1/4 tsp ground nutmeg (optional)
- 1/4 tsp salt

For the Crumble Topping:

- 1/2 cup rolled oats
- 1/4 cup almond flour
- 1/4 cup chopped nuts (walnuts, pecans, or almonds)
- 1/4 cup honey or maple syrup
- 1/4 cup coconut oil, melted
- 1/2 tsp ground cinnamon
- 1/4 tsp salt
- Non-stick spray

Instructions:

1. For three minutes, preheat the air fryer to 350°F (175°C).
2. Put the apple slices, lemon juice, honey, maple syrup, grated nutmeg (if using), ground cinnamon, and salt in a large mixing basin. Toss to evenly coat the apples.

3. Lightly mist a baking dish that fits into the basket of your air fryer that is suitable for the oven with non-stick spray.

4. Evenly distribute the apple mixture into the baking dish that has been preheated.

5. Transfer the rolled oats, almond flour, chopped nuts, melted coconut oil, ground cinnamon, honey or maple syrup, and salt to a different mixing bowl. Mix until crumbly and all of the ingredients are properly incorporated.

6. Evenly top the apple mixture with the crumble topping.

7. Insert the baking dish into the basket of the air fryer.

8. Air fry for 15 to 20 minutes at 350°F/175°C, or until the apples are soft and the crumble topping is browned. Midway through the cooking time, check and make any required adjustments.

9. Before serving, carefully take the baking dish out of the air fryer and allow the apple-oat crumble to cool for a few minutes.

10. Serve warm, with the option to add some Greek yogurt or vanilla ice cream on top.

Nutritional Information (per serving, based on 6 servings):

- **Calories: 220**
- **Protein: 2g**

- **Carbohydrates: 38g**
- **Dietary Fiber: 5g**
- **Sugars: 25g**
- **Total Fat: 8g**
- **Saturated Fat: 5g**
- **Sodium: 100mg**
- **Potassium: 250mg**

9. Air Fryer Stuffed Dates

Ingredients:

- 12 Medjool dates
- 1/4 cup almond butter or peanut butter
- 1/4 cup chopped nuts (walnuts, pecans, or almonds)
- 1/4 tsp ground cinnamon
- 1 tsp honey or maple syrup (optional)
- Non-stick spray

Instructions:

1. For three minutes, preheat the air fryer to 350°F (175°C).
2. Remove the pit from each date by carefully cutting it lengthwise.
3. Combine the ground cinnamon, chopped nuts, and almond or peanut butter in a small bowl. For

added sweetness, feel free to use honey or maple syrup.

4. Press the edges of each date gently closed after stuffing them with roughly a spoonful of the nut butter mixture.

5. Lightly mist the nonstick spray on the air fryer basket.

6. Arrange the packed dates in a single layer within the air fryer basket.

7. Air fry for 5 to 7 minutes at 350°F/175°C, or until the dates are heated through and have a hint of caramelization.

8. Before serving, carefully take the dates out of the air fryer and let them cool for a few minutes.

9. As a sweet dessert, serve warm.

Nutritional Information (per serving, based on 12 stuffed dates):

- **Calories: 100**
- **Protein: 2g**
- **Carbohydrates: 18g**
- **Dietary Fiber: 3g**
- **Sugars: 14g**
- **Total Fat: 3g**
- **Saturated Fat: 0.5g**
- **Sodium: 2mg**
- **Potassium: 180mg**

10. Air Fryer Peach Cobbler Cups

Ingredients:

For the Filling:

- 3 medium peaches, peeled, pitted, and sliced
- 1 tbsp lemon juice
- 1/4 cup honey or maple syrup
- 1 tsp ground cinnamon
- 1/4 tsp ground nutmeg (optional)
- 1/4 tsp salt

For the Crumble Topping:

- 1/2 cup rolled oats
- 1/4 cup almond flour
- 1/4 cup chopped nuts (walnuts, pecans, or almonds)
- 1/4 cup honey or maple syrup
- 1/4 cup coconut oil, melted
- 1/2 tsp ground cinnamon
- 1/4 tsp salt
- Non-stick spray

Instructions:

1. For three minutes, preheat the air fryer to 350°F (175°C).

2. Put the peach slices, lemon juice, honey, maple syrup, grated nutmeg (if using), ground cinnamon, and salt in a large mixing basin. Toss to evenly coat the peaches.

3. Lightly use non-stick spray to coat four to six tiny oven-safe ramekins or baking cups.

4. Evenly divide the peach mixture among the ramekins that have been made.

5. Transfer the rolled oats, almond flour, chopped almonds, melted coconut oil, ground cinnamon, honey or maple syrup, and salt to a different mixing bowl. Mix until crumbly and all of the ingredients are properly incorporated.

6. Evenly cover the peach mixture in each ramekin with crumble topping.

7. Make sure the ramekins are not in contact with one another when you place them in the air fryer basket.

8. Air fry the peaches for 12 to 15 minutes at 350°F/175°C, or until they are soft and the crumble topping is golden brown. Midway through the cooking time, check and make any required adjustments.

9. Before serving, carefully take the ramekins out of the air fryer and allow the peach cobbler cups to cool for a few minutes.

10. Serve warm, with the option to add some Greek yogurt or vanilla ice cream on top.

Nutritional Information (per serving, based on 6 servings):

- **Calories: 200**
- **Protein: 3g**
- **Carbohydrates: 32g**
- **Dietary Fiber: 4g**
- **Sugars: 18g**
- **Total Fat: 8g**
- **Saturated Fat: 5g**
- **Sodium: 80mg**
- **Potassium: 250mg**

CHAPTER EIGHT: FLAVORFUL KIDNEY TRANSPLANT AIR FRYER SEVEN DAY MEAL PLAN

Using your air fryer, you can enjoy tasty, kidney-friendly meals with this seven-day meal plan. With an emphasis on simple preparation and balanced nutrition, each meal has been thoughtfully created to satisfy the dietary requirements of kidney transplant patients. You may discover satisfying and healthful breakfast, lunch, and dinner alternatives with this meal plan that will aid in your recuperation. Enjoy these quick and filling meals as you go on a healthier eating journey!

Day 1

Breakfast: Air Fryer Apple Chips with Greek Yogurt

Ingredients:

- 2 medium apples (any variety)
- 1/2 tsp ground cinnamon
- 1/4 tsp ground nutmeg (optional)
- Non-stick spray
- 1 cup Greek yogurt (plain or flavored)

Instructions:

1. Set the air fryer's temperature for three minutes at 300°F (150°C).
2. Peel, core, and wash the apples. The apples should be finely sliced into rounds that are about 1/8 inch thick using a mandoline or sharp knife.
3. Make sure the apple slices are equally covered by tossing them in a big mixing basin with ground nutmeg (if using) and cinnamon.
4. Lightly mist the nonstick spray on the air fryer basket. Make sure the apple slices do not overlap as you arrange them in the air fryer basket in a single layer. Cooking them in batches might be necessary to prevent crowding.
5. Air fried the slices for 15 to 20 minutes at 300°F (150°C), turning them halfway through. Observe

them closely to avoid burning them. The apple slices ought to be crispy and golden brown.

6. Carefully take the apple chips out of the air fryer and set them on a wire rack to cool until they are crispy and faintly browned. When they cool, they will keep getting crispier.

7. Serve the apple chips with a side of Greek yogurt for dipping. The creamy yogurt complements the sweet and crispy apple chips perfectly.

Nutritional Information (per serving, based on 4 servings):

- **Calories: 100**
- **Protein: 6g**
- **Carbohydrates: 20g**
- **Dietary Fiber: 3g**
- **Sugars: 12g**
- **Total Fat: 2g**
- **Saturated Fat: 1g**
- **Sodium: 30mg**
- **Potassium: 220mg**

Lunch: Air Fryer Quinoa-Stuffed Bell Peppers

Ingredients:

- 4 medium bell peppers (any color)
- 1 cup cooked quinoa
- 1/2 cup canned black beans, rinsed and drained
- 1/2 cup corn kernels (fresh, frozen, or canned)
- 1 small onion, finely chopped
- 1 clove garlic, minced
- 1 teaspoon ground cumin
- 1 teaspoon chili powder
- 1/2 teaspoon paprika
- 1/4 teaspoon salt (optional, check with your dietitian)
- 1/4 teaspoon ground black pepper
- 1/2 cup shredded low-fat cheese (optional, check with your dietitian)
- Fresh cilantro for garnish (optional)
- Olive oil spray

Instructions:

1. Slice off the bell peppers' tops, then take out the seeds and membranes. Put aside.
2. Put the cooked quinoa, black beans, corn, chopped onion, minced garlic, ground cumin, paprika, chili powder, salt, and black pepper in a big bowl. Blend thoroughly until everything is properly integrated.
3. Gently press down to firmly put the quinoa mixture inside each bell pepper.

4. Top each filled pepper with a little quantity of cheese, if using.

5. Set your air fryer's temperature for three to five minutes at 360°F (180°C).

6. To keep the air fryer basket from sticking, lightly mist it with olive oil spray.

7. Holding the filled bell peppers upright, place them in the air fryer basket. The number of batches you need to cook them in will depend on how big your air fryer is.

8. Simmer for ten to fifteen minutes, or until the filling is well cooked and the peppers are soft. If cheese is being used, it must be bubbling and melted.

9. Using tongs, carefully take the bell peppers out of the air fryer.

10. Before serving, allow them to cool somewhat.

11. If preferred, garnish with fresh cilantro.

Nutritional Information (per stuffed pepper, without cheese):

- **Calories: 150**
- **Protein: 5g**
- **Carbohydrates: 30g**
- **Dietary Fiber: 6g**
- **Sugars: 5g**
- **Fat: 1.5g**
- **Sodium: 120mg (varies with salt content)**

- **Potassium: 500mg**
- **Phosphorus: 100mg**

Dinner: Air Fryer Lentil-Stuffed Portobello Mushrooms

Ingredients:

- 4 large portobello mushrooms, stems removed and gills scraped out
- 1 cup cooked lentils
- 1 small onion, finely chopped
- 1 small red bell pepper, finely chopped
- 1 clove garlic, minced
- 1/4 cup whole wheat breadcrumbs
- 1/4 cup grated Parmesan cheese (optional, check with your dietitian)
- 1 tablespoon fresh parsley, chopped (optional)
- 1 tablespoon olive oil
- 1 teaspoon Italian seasoning
- 1/4 teaspoon ground black pepper
- 1/4 teaspoon salt (optional, check with your dietitian)
- Olive oil spray

Instructions:

1. Set your air fryer's temperature for three to five minutes at 375°F (190°C).

2. Heat the olive oil in a big skillet over medium heat. Add the minced garlic, red bell pepper, and diced onion. Sauté for approximately five minutes, or until the veggies are tender.

3. Fill the skillet with the cooked lentils, Italian spice, black pepper, and salt (if using). After combining, cook for a further two to three minutes. Take off the heat.

4. Add the grated Parmesan cheese (if using) and whole wheat breadcrumbs to the lentil mixture. Blend thoroughly until everything is properly integrated.

5. Lightly mist both sides of the portobello mushroom caps with olive oil spray.

6. Spoon the lentil mixture into each mushroom cap, lightly pushing to compact the filling.

7. Arrange the filled mushrooms in a single layer within the air fryer basket. The number of batches you need to cook them in will depend on how big your air fryer is.

8. Cook for ten to twelve minutes, or until the filling is well cooked and has a hint of crunch on top, and the mushrooms are soft.

9. Using tongs, carefully take the stuffed mushrooms out of the air fryer.

10. Before serving, allow them to cool somewhat.

11. If preferred, garnish with fresh parsley.

Nutritional Information (per stuffed mushroom, based on 4 servings):

- **Calories: 180**
- **Protein: 9g**
- **Carbohydrates: 23g**
- **Dietary Fiber: 7g**
- **Sugars: 5g**
- **Fat: 6g**
- **Sodium: 220mg (varies with salt and cheese content)**
- **Potassium: 700mg**
- **Phosphorus: 140mg**

Day 2

Breakfast: Air Fryer Banana Chips with Almond Butter

Ingredients:

- 2 ripe but firm bananas
- 1 tbsp lemon juice

- 1 tbsp water
- Non-stick spray
- 1/2 cup almond butter (smooth or chunky)

Instructions:

1. Preheat the air fryer to 300°F (150°C) for 3 minutes.
2. In a small bowl, mix the lemon juice and water.
3. Peel the bananas and slice them thinly, about 1/8 inch thick.
4. Lightly dip each banana slice in the lemon juice mixture to prevent browning.
5. Lightly spray the air fryer basket with non-stick spray.
6. Place the banana slices in the air fryer basket in a single layer, ensuring they do not overlap. You may need to cook them in batches to avoid overcrowding.
7. Air fry at 300°F (150°C) for 15-20 minutes, flipping the slices halfway through the cooking time. Keep a close eye on them to prevent burning.
8. Once the banana chips are golden brown and crispy, carefully remove them from the air fryer and place them on a wire rack to cool. They will continue to crisp up as they cool.
9. Allow the banana chips to cool completely to ensure maximum crispiness.

10. Serve the banana chips with a side of almond butter for dipping or spreading.

Nutritional Information (per serving, based on 4 servings):

- **Calories: 160**
- **Protein: 4g**
- **Carbohydrates: 22g**
- **Dietary Fiber: 4g**
- **Sugars: 12g**
- **Total Fat: 7g**
- **Saturated Fat: 0.5g**
- **Sodium: 0mg**
- **Potassium: 300mg**

Lunch: Chickpea and Veggie Patties with a Side Salad

Ingredients:

For the Chickpea and Veggie Patties:

- 1 can (15 oz) chickpeas, drained and rinsed
- 1/2 cup grated carrots
- 1/2 cup finely chopped spinach
- 1/4 cup finely diced red bell pepper

- 1/4 cup finely chopped onion
- 2 cloves garlic, minced
- 1/4 cup whole wheat breadcrumbs
- 1 large egg
- 1 tbsp olive oil
- 1 tsp ground cumin
- 1/2 tsp paprika
- 1/4 tsp black pepper
- 1/4 tsp salt
- Non-stick spray

For the Side Salad:

- 4 cups mixed greens (spinach, arugula, and lettuce)
- 1/2 cup cherry tomatoes, halved
- 1/4 cup cucumber, sliced
- 1/4 cup red onion, thinly sliced
- 1/4 cup shredded carrots
- 2 tbsp olive oil
- 1 tbsp balsamic vinegar
- 1 tsp Dijon mustard
- Salt and black pepper to taste

Instructions:

1. Preheat the air fryer to 375°F (190°C) for 3 minutes.

2. In a large mixing bowl, mash the chickpeas with a fork or potato masher until mostly smooth.

3. Add the grated carrots, chopped spinach, diced red bell pepper, chopped onion, minced garlic, whole wheat breadcrumbs, and egg to the mashed chickpeas. Mix until well combined.

4. Add the olive oil, ground cumin, paprika, black pepper, and salt to the mixture. Stir to incorporate all the ingredients evenly.

5. Shape the mixture into 8 patties, about 1/2 inch thick.

6. Lightly spray the air fryer basket with non-stick spray. Place the patties in the basket in a single layer. You may need to cook them in batches to avoid overcrowding.

7. Air fry the patties at 375°F (190°C) for 10-12 minutes, flipping halfway through, until they are golden brown and crispy.

8. While the patties are cooking, prepare the side salad. In a large bowl, combine the mixed greens, cherry tomatoes, cucumber, red onion, and shredded carrots.

9. In a small bowl, whisk together the olive oil, balsamic vinegar, Dijon mustard, salt, and black pepper to make the dressing.

10. Pour the dressing over the salad and toss to combine.

11. Once the patties are done, carefully remove them from the air fryer and let them cool for a few minutes.

12. Serve the chickpea and veggie patties warm alongside the side salad.

Nutritional Information (per serving, based on 4 servings):

- **Calories: 300**
- **Protein: 10g**
- **Carbohydrates: 30g**
- **Dietary Fiber: 8g**
- **Sugars: 6g**
- **Total Fat: 15g**
- **Saturated Fat: 2g**
- **Sodium: 400mg**
- **Potassium: 700mg**

Dinner: Air Fryer Sweet Potato and Black Bean Burritos

Ingredients:

- 2 medium sweet potatoes, peeled and diced
- 1 can (15 oz) black beans, rinsed and drained
- 1 small red onion, finely chopped

- 1 small red bell pepper, diced
- 1 clove garlic, minced
- 1 teaspoon ground cumin
- 1 teaspoon chili powder
- 1/2 teaspoon smoked paprika
- 1/4 teaspoon ground black pepper
- 1/4 teaspoon salt (optional, check with your dietitian)
- 1 tablespoon olive oil
- 1/4 cup fresh cilantro, chopped (optional)
- 4 large whole wheat tortillas
- 1/2 cup shredded low-fat cheese (optional, check with your dietitian)
- Olive oil spray

For Serving:

- Salsa (optional, check with your dietitian)
- Avocado slices (optional, check with your dietitian)
- Lime wedges

Instructions:

1. Set your air fryer's temperature for three to five minutes at 375°F (190°C).
2. Combine the diced sweet potatoes, black pepper, smoked paprika, chili powder, ground cumin, and

olive oil in a big bowl. Toss until the potatoes are uniformly coated.

3. To keep the air fryer basket from sticking, lightly mist it with olive oil spray.

4. Arrange the seasoned sweet potatoes in a single layer within the air fryer basket. Sweet potatoes should be cooked for 15 to 20 minutes, shaking the basket halfway through, or until they are soft and beginning to crisp up.

5. In a sizable mixing basin, mix the black beans, minced garlic, diced red bell pepper, chopped onion, and chopped cilantro (if using) while the sweet potatoes are cooking.

6. Add the cooked sweet potatoes to the black bean mixture and gently toss to incorporate.

7. To make the tortillas more malleable, briefly reheat them in the microwave or on the stovetop.

8. Fill the middle of each tortilla with some of the sweet potato and black bean mixture. If using, top with shredded cheese.

9. To create a burrito, carefully roll up each tortilla, tucking in the edges as you roll.

10. Reapply a little coat of olive oil spray to the air fryer basket. Put the burritos into the air fryer basket, seam side down. The number of batches you need to cook them in will depend on how big your air fryer is.

11. Gently mist the burritos' tops with olive oil spray.

12. Bake the burritos in the air fryer for 5 to 7 minutes, or until the tortillas are crispy and golden brown, at 375°F (190°C).

13. Using tongs, carefully take the burritos out of the air fryer.

14. Allow them to cool somewhat before serving, if you'd like, with avocado slices, salsa, and lime wedges.

Nutritional Information (per burrito, based on 4 burritos):

- **Calories: 350**
- **Protein: 10g**
- **Carbohydrates: 60g**
- **Dietary Fiber: 12g**
- **Sugars: 7g**
- **Fat: 9g**
- **Sodium: 400mg (varies with salt and cheese content)**
- **Potassium: 700mg**
- **Phosphorus: 150mg**

Day 3

Breakfast: Air Fryer Pear Slices with Cinnamon

Ingredients:

- 2 ripe pears
- 1 tsp ground cinnamon
- 1/2 tsp ground nutmeg (optional)
- 1 tsp honey or maple syrup (optional)
- Non-stick spray

Instructions:

1. For three minutes, preheat the air fryer to 350°F (175°C).
2. Give the pears a wash and core. Cut them into wedges that are just 1/4 inch thick.
3. Gently toss the pear slices with ground nutmeg (if using) and cinnamon in a large mixing dish until they are well coated. For added sweetness, feel free to drizzle with honey or maple syrup and toss to coat.
4. Lightly mist the nonstick spray on the air fryer basket.
5. Make sure the pear slices do not overlap when you arrange them in the air fryer basket in a single layer. Cooking them in batches might be necessary to prevent crowding.

6. Air fry the pear slices for 8 to 10 minutes at 350°F (175°C), turning them halfway through, or until they are soft and have a hint of caramel.

7. Before serving, gently take the cooked pear slices out of the air fryer and let them cool for a few minutes.

8. Savor the warm dessert right away.

Nutritional Information (per serving, based on 4 servings):

- **Calories: 60**
- **Protein: 0.5g**
- **Carbohydrates: 16g**
- **Dietary Fiber: 3g**
- **Sugars: 10g**
- **Total Fat: 0.2g**
- **Saturated Fat: 0g**
- **Sodium: 0mg**
- **Potassium: 120mg**

Lunch: Air Fryer Tofu and Veggie Stir-Fry with Brown Rice

Ingredients:

For the Tofu and Veggie Stir-Fry:

- 1 block (14 oz) firm tofu, drained and pressed
- 2 cups broccoli florets
- 1 red bell pepper, sliced
- 1 small carrot, julienned
- 1 small onion, sliced
- 2 cloves garlic, minced
- 2 tbsp low-sodium soy sauce
- 1 tbsp olive oil
- 1 tbsp cornstarch
- 1 tsp sesame oil (optional)
- 1/2 tsp ground ginger
- 1/4 tsp black pepper
- 1/4 tsp red pepper flakes (optional)

For the Brown Rice:

- 1 cup brown rice
- 2 cups water or low-sodium vegetable broth

For Garnish:

- Fresh sesame seeds
- Chopped green onions

Instructions:

1. Cook the brown rice by combining 1 cup of brown rice and 2 cups of water or vegetable broth in

a saucepan. Bring to a boil, then reduce heat to low, cover, and simmer for about 45 minutes or until the rice is tender and the liquid is absorbed. Remove from heat and let it sit, covered, for 10 minutes, then fluff with a fork.

2. Preheat the air fryer to 375°F (190°C) for 3 minutes.

3. Cut the pressed tofu into 1-inch cubes. In a large bowl, toss the tofu cubes with cornstarch until they are evenly coated.

4. Lightly spray the air fryer basket with non-stick spray. Place the tofu cubes in the basket in a single layer.

5. Air fry the tofu at 375°F (190°C) for 12-15 minutes, shaking the basket halfway through, until the tofu is golden and crispy.

6. While the tofu is cooking, prepare the vegetables. In a large mixing bowl, combine the broccoli florets, sliced red bell pepper, julienned carrot, sliced onion, and minced garlic.

7. In a small bowl, mix together the low-sodium soy sauce, olive oil, sesame oil (if using), ground ginger, black pepper, and red pepper flakes (if using).

8. Pour the soy sauce mixture over the vegetables and toss to coat evenly.

9. Once the tofu is done, remove it from the air fryer and set it aside.

10. Place the seasoned vegetables in the air fryer basket. Air fry at 375°F (190°C) for 10-12 minutes, shaking the basket halfway through, until the vegetables are tender but still crisp.

11. Combine the cooked tofu with the vegetables in the air fryer basket and air fry for an additional 2-3 minutes to heat everything through and combine flavors.

12. Remove the tofu and vegetable stir-fry from the air fryer and serve over the cooked brown rice.

13. Garnish with fresh sesame seeds and chopped green onions if desired.

Nutritional Information (per serving, based on 4 servings):

- **Calories: 350**
- **Protein: 13g**
- **Carbohydrates: 45g**
- **Dietary Fiber: 6g**
- **Sugars: 5g**
- **Total Fat: 14g**
- **Saturated Fat: 2g**
- **Sodium: 400mg**
- **Potassium: 500mg**

Dinner: Air Fryer Eggplant and Chickpea Curry with Whole Grain Naan

Ingredients:

For the Eggplant and Chickpea Curry:

- 1 large eggplant, diced
- 1 can (15 oz) chickpeas, drained and rinsed
- 1 medium onion, diced
- 2 cloves garlic, minced
- 1-inch piece of ginger, grated
- 1 can (14 oz) diced tomatoes
- 1 cup coconut milk
- 2 tbsp olive oil
- 1 tbsp curry powder
- 1 tsp ground cumin
- 1 tsp ground coriander
- 1/2 tsp turmeric
- 1/2 tsp paprika
- 1/4 tsp cayenne pepper (optional)
- 1/4 tsp salt
- 1/4 tsp black pepper
- Fresh cilantro for garnish

For the Whole Grain Naan:

- 2 cups whole wheat flour

- 1/2 cup plain Greek yogurt
- 1/4 cup warm water
- 1 tbsp olive oil
- 1 tsp baking powder
- 1/2 tsp salt

Instructions:

1. Preheat the air fryer to 375°F (190°C) for 3 minutes.

2. In a large bowl, toss the diced eggplant with 1 tbsp of olive oil, salt, and black pepper until evenly coated.

3. Lightly spray the air fryer basket with non-stick spray. Place the eggplant in the basket in a single layer.

4. Air fry the eggplant at 375°F (190°C) for 15-20 minutes, shaking the basket halfway through, until the eggplant is tender and slightly crispy.

5. While the eggplant is cooking, heat 1 tbsp of olive oil in a large skillet over medium heat. Add the diced onion, minced garlic, and grated ginger, sautéing until the onion is translucent, about 3-4 minutes.

6. Add the curry powder, ground cumin, ground coriander, turmeric, paprika, and cayenne pepper (if using) to the skillet. Stir to combine and cook for 1-2 minutes until fragrant.

7. Add the diced tomatoes and coconut milk to the skillet, stirring to combine. Bring to a simmer.

8. Once the eggplant is done, add it to the skillet along with the chickpeas. Stir to combine and simmer for an additional 10 minutes, allowing the flavors to meld.

9. While the curry is simmering, prepare the whole grain naan. In a large mixing bowl, combine the whole wheat flour, Greek yogurt, warm water, olive oil, baking powder, and salt. Mix until a dough forms.

10. Divide the dough into 6 equal pieces and roll each piece into a ball. Flatten each ball into a round or oval shape about 1/4 inch thick.

11. Preheat a skillet or griddle over medium-high heat. Cook each naan for 2-3 minutes on each side until golden brown and puffed up.

12. Serve the eggplant and chickpea curry garnished with fresh cilantro, alongside the warm whole grain naan.

Nutritional Information (per serving, based on 6 servings):

- **Calories: 350**
- **Protein: 10g**
- **Carbohydrates: 45g**
- **Dietary Fiber: 10g**
- **Sugars: 7g**

- Total Fat: 14g
- Saturated Fat: 4.5g
- Sodium: 400mg
- Potassium: 750mg

Day 4

Breakfast: Air Fryer Oatmeal Cookies with a Glass of Milk

Ingredients:

- 1 cup rolled oats
- 1/2 cup whole wheat flour
- 1/2 cup unsweetened applesauce
- 1/4 cup honey or maple syrup
- 1/4 cup coconut oil, melted
- 1/4 cup raisins or dried cranberries
- 1/4 cup chopped nuts (walnuts or almonds)
- 1 tsp vanilla extract
- 1 tsp ground cinnamon
- 1/2 tsp baking powder
- 1/4 tsp salt
- Non-stick spray
- 2 cups milk (dairy or plant-based)

Instructions:

1. Preheat the air fryer to 350°F (175°C) for 3 minutes.

2. In a large mixing bowl, combine the rolled oats, whole wheat flour, ground cinnamon, baking powder, and salt. Mix well.

3. In another bowl, whisk together the unsweetened applesauce, honey or maple syrup, melted coconut oil, and vanilla extract until well combined.

4. Pour the wet ingredients into the dry ingredients and stir until just combined.

5. Fold in the raisins or dried cranberries and chopped nuts.

6. Line the air fryer basket with parchment paper to prevent the cookies from sticking.

7. Scoop out tablespoon-sized portions of the dough and place them on the parchment paper, flattening them slightly with your fingers. Leave some space between the cookies as they will spread slightly during cooking.

8. Air fry at 350°F (175°C) for 8-10 minutes, or until the cookies are golden brown and set. Check the cookies halfway through the cooking time and adjust if necessary.

9. Carefully remove the cookies from the air fryer and let them cool on a wire rack.

10. Pour the milk into glasses while the cookies are cooling.

11. Serve the oatmeal cookies with a glass of milk for a delicious and nutritious snack or dessert.

Nutritional Information (per serving, based on 12 cookies without milk):

- **Calories: 110**
- **Protein: 2g**
- **Carbohydrates: 15g**
- **Dietary Fiber: 2g**
- **Sugars: 7g**
- **Total Fat: 5g**
- **Saturated Fat: 3g**
- **Sodium: 50mg**
- **Potassium: 80mg**

Lunch: Sweet Potato and Black Bean Tacos

Ingredients:

- 2 medium sweet potatoes, peeled and diced
- 1 can (15 oz) black beans, rinsed and drained
- 1 small red onion, diced
- 1 small red bell pepper, diced

- 1 tablespoon olive oil
- 1 teaspoon ground cumin
- 1/2 teaspoon chili powder
- 1/2 teaspoon paprika
- 1/4 teaspoon ground black pepper
- 1/4 teaspoon salt (optional, check with your dietitian)
- 8 small corn tortillas
- Fresh cilantro for garnish (optional)
- Lime wedges for serving (optional)

Instructions:

1. Set your air fryer's temperature for three to five minutes at 375°F (190°C).
2. Place the diced sweet potatoes in a big basin and toss them until they are uniformly coated with olive oil, ground cumin, chili powder, paprika, black pepper, and salt (if using).
3. To keep the air fryer basket from sticking, lightly mist it with olive oil spray.
4. Arrange the seasoned sweet potatoes in a single layer within the air fryer basket. Sweet potatoes should be cooked for 15 to 20 minutes, shaking the basket halfway through, or until they are soft and beginning to crisp up.
5. In a medium-sized dish, mix the diced red onion, diced red bell pepper, and black beans while the sweet potatoes are cooking. Put aside.

6. Carefully take the sweet potatoes out of the air fryer and combine them with the black bean mixture. Gently toss to mix.

7. Use the air fryer to reheat the corn tortillas for one to two minutes, or until they are soft and malleable.

8. Spoon the black bean and sweet potato mixture onto each tortilla to assemble the tacos.

9. If preferred, garnish with fresh cilantro and serve with lime wedges.

Nutritional Information (per taco):

- **Calories: 120**
- **Protein: 3g**
- **Carbohydrates: 23g**
- **Dietary Fiber: 5g**
- **Sugars: 3g**
- **Fat: 3g**
- **Sodium: 150mg (varies with salt content)**
- **Potassium: 350mg**
- **Phosphorus: 60mg**

Dinner: Air Fryer Barley and Vegetable Casserole

Ingredients:

- 1 cup pearl barley
- 2 cups low-sodium vegetable broth
- 1/2 cup diced carrots
- 1/2 cup diced bell peppers (any color)
- 1/2 cup diced zucchini
- 1/2 cup diced onions
- 1/2 cup chopped broccoli florets
- 2 cloves garlic, minced
- 1 tsp dried thyme
- 1 tsp dried oregano
- 1/2 tsp ground black pepper
- 1/4 tsp salt
- 1 tbsp olive oil
- 1/4 cup grated Parmesan cheese (optional)
- Non-stick spray

Instructions:

1. Follow the directions on the package to cook the pearl barley in the low-sodium vegetable broth. Usually, this takes between 25 and 30 minutes. After cooking, place it aside.
2. Set the air fryer's temperature for three minutes to 350°F/175°C.
3. Add the chopped broccoli florets, bell peppers, zucchini, onions, and diced carrots to a large mixing bowl.

4. Combine the vegetable combination with the minced garlic, olive oil, salt, crushed black pepper, dried thyme, and dried oregano. Toss until the oil and spices are distributed equally over the veggies.

5. Use a little amount of nonstick spray to coat a casserole dish or oven-safe baking dish that fits within the air fryer basket.

6. Evenly distribute the cooked barley across the casserole dish.

7. Evenly spoon the seasoned vegetable mixture over the barley on top of it.

8. To keep the veggies from drying out, cover the casserole dish with aluminum foil.

9. Insert the casserole dish into the basket of the air fryer.

10. Air fried the veggies for 20 to 25 minutes, or until they are soft, at 350°F/175°C.

11. Take off the foil and sprinkle the Parmesan cheese on top of the casserole, if using. Put the dish back in the air fryer and let it cook for a further three to five minutes, or until the cheese is bubbling and melted.

12. Before serving, carefully take the casserole dish out of the air fryer and allow it to cool for a few minutes.

Nutritional Information (per serving, based on 6 servings without Parmesan cheese):

- **Calories: 200**
- **Protein: 5g**
- **Carbohydrates: 38g**
- **Dietary Fiber: 7g**
- **Sugars: 4g**
- **Total Fat: 4g**
- **Saturated Fat: 0.5g**
- **Sodium: 250mg**
- **Potassium: 300mg**

Day 5

Breakfast: Air Fryer Apple Oat Crumble

Ingredients:

For the Filling:

- 4 medium apples (any variety), peeled, cored, and sliced
- 1 tbsp lemon juice
- 1/4 cup honey or maple syrup
- 1 tsp ground cinnamon
- 1/4 tsp ground nutmeg (optional)
- 1/4 tsp salt

For the Crumble Topping:

- 1/2 cup rolled oats
- 1/4 cup almond flour
- 1/4 cup chopped nuts (walnuts, pecans, or almonds)
- 1/4 cup honey or maple syrup
- 1/4 cup coconut oil, melted
- 1/2 tsp ground cinnamon
- 1/4 tsp salt
- Non-stick spray

Instructions:

1. For three minutes, preheat the air fryer to 350°F (175°C).
2. Put the apple slices, lemon juice, honey, maple syrup, grated nutmeg (if using), ground cinnamon, and salt in a large mixing basin. Toss to evenly coat the apples.
3. Lightly mist a baking dish that fits into the basket of your air fryer that is suitable for the oven with non-stick spray.
4. Evenly distribute the apple mixture into the baking dish that has been preheated.
5. Transfer the rolled oats, almond flour, chopped nuts, melted coconut oil, ground cinnamon, honey or maple syrup, and salt to a different mixing bowl.

Mix until crumbly and all of the ingredients are properly incorporated.

6. Evenly top the apple mixture with the crumble topping.

7. Insert the baking dish into the basket of the air fryer.

8. Air fry for 15 to 20 minutes at 350°F/175°C, or until the apples are soft and the crumble topping is browned. Midway through the cooking time, check and make any required adjustments.

9. Before serving, carefully take the baking dish out of the air fryer and allow the apple-oat crumble to cool for a few minutes.

10. Serve warm, with the option to add some Greek yogurt or vanilla ice cream on top.

Nutritional Information (per serving, based on 6 servings):

- **Calories: 220**
- **Protein: 2g**
- **Carbohydrates: 38g**
- **Dietary Fiber: 5g**
- **Sugars: 25g**
- **Total Fat: 8g**
- **Saturated Fat: 5g**
- **Sodium: 100mg**
- **Potassium: 250mg**

Lunch: Cauliflower and Lentil Rice Bowls

Ingredients:

- 1 medium head of cauliflower, cut into florets
- 1 cup cooked lentils (brown or green)
- 1 cup cooked brown rice
- 1 small red bell pepper, diced
- 1 small cucumber, diced
- 1 small carrot, grated
- 1/4 cup red onion, finely chopped
- 1 tablespoon olive oil
- 1 teaspoon ground cumin
- 1/2 teaspoon smoked paprika
- 1/4 teaspoon ground black pepper
- 1/4 teaspoon salt (optional, check with your dietitian)
- 1 tablespoon fresh parsley or cilantro, chopped (optional)
- Lemon wedges for serving (optional)

Instructions:

1. Set your air fryer's temperature for three to five minutes at 375°F (190°C).
2. Place the cauliflower florets in a big basin and toss them until they are uniformly coated with olive

oil, smoked paprika, ground cumin, black pepper, and salt (if using).

3. To keep the air fryer basket from sticking, lightly mist it with olive oil spray.

4. Arrange the seasoned cauliflower florets in a single layer within the air fryer basket. Cook, shaking the basket halfway through, until the cauliflower is soft and beginning to crisp up, 12 to 15 minutes.

5. Prepare the remaining ingredients while the cauliflower cooks. The cooked lentils, cooked brown rice, sliced cucumber, diced bell pepper, shredded carrot, and chopped red onion should all be combined in a big bowl. Gently toss to mix.

6. Carefully take the cauliflower out of the air fryer and add it to the bowl containing the rice and lentil mixture. Gently toss to mix.

7. Transfer the mixture into dishes and, if preferred, top with cilantro or fresh parsley.

8. For an additional taste explosion, serve with lemon slices on the side.

Nutritional Information (per serving, based on 4 servings):

- **Calories: 220**
- **Protein: 8g**
- **Carbohydrates: 35g**
- **Dietary Fiber: 10g**

- Sugars: 5g
- Fat: 5g
- Sodium: 150mg (varies with salt content)
- Potassium: 600mg
- Phosphorus: 150mg

Dinner: Air Fryer Broccoli and Tofu Stir-Fry with Quinoa

Ingredients:

- 1 block (14 oz) firm tofu, drained and pressed
- 2 cups broccoli florets
- 1 red bell pepper, sliced
- 1 small onion, sliced
- 2 cloves garlic, minced
- 2 tbsp low-sodium soy sauce
- 1 tbsp olive oil
- 1 tbsp cornstarch
- 1 tsp sesame oil (optional)
- 1/2 tsp ground ginger
- 1/4 tsp black pepper
- 1/4 tsp red pepper flakes (optional)
- 1 cup cooked quinoa
- Fresh sesame seeds and green onions for garnish (optional)
- Non-stick spray

Instructions:

1. Preheat the air fryer to 375°F (190°C) for 3 minutes.

2. Cut the pressed tofu into 1-inch cubes.

3. In a large bowl, toss the tofu cubes with cornstarch, ensuring they are evenly coated.

4. Lightly spray the air fryer basket with non-stick spray. Place the tofu cubes in the basket in a single layer.

5. Air fry the tofu at 375°F (190°C) for 12-15 minutes, shaking the basket halfway through, until the tofu is golden and crispy.

6. While the tofu is cooking, prepare the vegetables. In a large mixing bowl, combine the broccoli florets, sliced red bell pepper, sliced onion, and minced garlic.

7. In a small bowl, mix together the low-sodium soy sauce, olive oil, sesame oil (if using), ground ginger, black pepper, and red pepper flakes (if using).

8. Pour the soy sauce mixture over the vegetables and toss to coat evenly.

9. Once the tofu is done, remove it from the air fryer and set it aside.

10. Place the seasoned vegetables in the air fryer basket. Air fry at 375°F (190°C) for 10-12 minutes,

shaking the basket halfway through, until the vegetables are tender but still crisp.

11. Combine the cooked tofu with the vegetables in the air fryer basket and air fry for an additional 2-3 minutes to heat everything through and combine flavors.

12. Remove the stir-fry from the air fryer and serve over cooked quinoa.

13. Garnish with fresh sesame seeds and chopped green onions if desired.

Nutritional Information (per serving, based on 4 servings):

- **Calories: 300**
- **Protein: 14g**
- **Carbohydrates: 30g**
- **Dietary Fiber: 5g**
- **Sugars: 5g**
- **Total Fat: 14g**
- **Saturated Fat: 2g**
- **Sodium: 400mg**
- **Potassium: 600mg**

Day 6

Breakfast: Air Fryer Apple Chips with Peanut Butter

Ingredients:

- 2 medium apples (any variety)
- 1/2 tsp ground cinnamon
- 1/4 tsp ground nutmeg (optional)
- Non-stick spray
- 1/2 cup peanut butter (smooth or chunky)

Instructions:

1. Preheat the air fryer to 300°F (150°C) for 3 minutes.
2. Wash and core the apples. Using a mandoline or a sharp knife, thinly slice the apples into rounds about 1/8 inch thick.
3. In a large mixing bowl, toss the apple slices with ground cinnamon and ground nutmeg (if using), ensuring they are evenly coated.
4. Lightly spray the air fryer basket with non-stick spray.
5. Place the apple slices in the air fryer basket in a single layer, making sure they do not overlap. You may need to cook them in batches to avoid overcrowding.

6. Air fry at 300°F (150°C) for 15-20 minutes, flipping the slices halfway through the cooking time. Keep a close eye on them to prevent burning.

7. Once the apple slices are golden brown and crispy, carefully remove them from the air fryer and place them on a wire rack to cool. They will continue to crisp up as they cool.

8. Allow the apple chips to cool completely to ensure maximum crispiness.

9. Serve the apple chips with a side of peanut butter for dipping or spreading.

Nutritional Information (per serving, based on 4 servings):

- **Calories: 200**
- **Protein: 6g**
- **Carbohydrates: 27g**
- **Dietary Fiber: 5g**
- **Sugars: 17g**
- **Total Fat: 8g**
- **Saturated Fat: 1.5g**
- **Sodium: 80mg**
- **Potassium: 300mg**

Lunch: Air Fryer Stuffed Zucchini Boats

Ingredients:

- 4 medium zucchinis
- 1 cup cooked quinoa
- 1 can (15 oz) black beans, drained and rinsed
- 1/2 cup corn kernels (fresh, canned, or frozen)
- 1/2 cup diced tomatoes
- 1/2 cup shredded low-fat cheese (optional)
- 1 small onion, finely diced
- 2 cloves garlic, minced
- 1 tsp ground cumin
- 1/2 tsp chili powder
- 1/2 tsp paprika
- 1/4 tsp black pepper
- 1/4 tsp salt
- 1 tbsp olive oil
- Fresh cilantro for garnish (optional)
- Non-stick spray

Instructions:

1. Preheat the air fryer to 375°F (190°C) for 3 minutes.
2. Wash and halve the zucchinis lengthwise. Use a spoon to scoop out the seeds and flesh, creating a hollow center in each zucchini half.
3. Lightly spray the air fryer basket with non-stick spray.

4. Place the zucchini halves in the air fryer basket and air fry at 375°F (190°C) for 5 minutes to slightly soften them.

5. While the zucchinis are pre-cooking, heat olive oil in a skillet over medium heat. Add the diced onion and minced garlic, sautéing until they become translucent, about 3-4 minutes.

6. Add the cooked quinoa, black beans, corn kernels, diced tomatoes, ground cumin, chili powder, paprika, black pepper, and salt to the skillet. Stir to combine and cook for an additional 5 minutes.

7. Remove the zucchini halves from the air fryer and fill each one with the quinoa and vegetable mixture, pressing down lightly to pack the filling.

8. If using, sprinkle the shredded cheese evenly over the stuffed zucchinis.

9. Place the stuffed zucchinis back in the air fryer basket in a single layer.

10. Air fry at 375°F (190°C) for 8-10 minutes, or until the zucchinis are tender and the cheese is melted and bubbly.

11. Carefully remove the stuffed zucchinis from the air fryer and let them cool for a few minutes before serving.

12. Garnish with fresh cilantro if desired.

Nutritional Information (per serving, based on 4 servings without cheese):

- Calories: 180
- Protein: 6g
- Carbohydrates: 28g
- Dietary Fiber: 7g
- Sugars: 6g
- Total Fat: 6g
- Saturated Fat: 1g
- Sodium: 300mg
- Potassium: 700mg

Dinner: Air Fryer Quinoa and Veggie-Stuffed Tomatoes

Ingredients:

- 4 large tomatoes
- 1 cup cooked quinoa
- 1/2 cup canned black beans, rinsed and drained
- 1 small zucchini, finely diced
- 1 small red bell pepper, finely diced
- 1 small onion, finely chopped
- 1 clove garlic, minced
- 1 tablespoon olive oil
- 1 teaspoon ground cumin
- 1/2 teaspoon chili powder
- 1/4 teaspoon ground black pepper

- 1/4 teaspoon salt (optional, check with your dietitian)
- 1/4 cup grated Parmesan cheese (optional, check with your dietitian)
- Fresh parsley or cilantro for garnish (optional)

Instructions:

1. Set your air fryer's temperature for three to five minutes at 375°F (190°C).
2. Slice off the tops of the tomatoes and use a spoon to remove the insides, taking cautious not to pierce the outer walls. Remove the scooped-out meat and set aside the tomato tops.
3. Heat the olive oil in a big pan over medium heat. Add the red bell pepper, chopped onion, minced garlic, and cubed zucchini. Sauté for approximately five minutes, or until the veggies are tender.
4. Add the black beans, cooked quinoa, chili powder, ground cumin, black pepper, and salt (if needed). Cook for a further two to three minutes, or until well heated. Take off the heat.
5. Stuff the quinoa and vegetable mixture into each hollowed-out tomato, lightly pushing to compact the filling.
6. Top each filled tomato, if using, with a little pinch of grated Parmesan cheese.
7. To keep the air fryer basket from sticking, lightly mist it with olive oil spray.

8. Arrange the filled tomatoes in a single layer within the air fryer basket. The number of batches you need to cook them in will depend on how big your air fryer is.

9. Cook the stuffed tomatoes for 10 to 12 minutes, or until the tomatoes are soft and the filling is well cooked, at 375°F (190°C). If cheese is being used, it must be bubbling and melted.

10. Using tongs, carefully take the filled tomatoes out of the air fryer.

11. Before serving, let them cool somewhat.

12. If preferred, garnish with fresh cilantro or parsley.

Nutritional Information (per stuffed tomato, based on 4 servings):

- **Calories: 200**
- **Protein: 7g**
- **Carbohydrates: 28g**
- **Dietary Fiber: 6g**
- **Sugars: 8g**
- **Fat: 7g**
- **Sodium: 250mg (varies with salt and cheese content)**
- **Potassium: 600mg**
- **Phosphorus: 100mg**

Day 7

Breakfast: Air Fryer Banana Chips with a Smoothie

Ingredients:

For the Banana Chips:

- 2 ripe but firm bananas
- 1 tbsp lemon juice
- 1 tbsp water
- Non-stick spray

For the Smoothie:

- 1 cup frozen berries (strawberries, blueberries, or mixed)
- 1 banana
- 1/2 cup Greek yogurt
- 1 cup unsweetened almond milk (or any milk alternative)
- 1 tbsp honey or maple syrup (optional)

Instructions:

1. Preheat the air fryer to 300°F (150°C) for 3 minutes.

2. In a small bowl, mix the lemon juice and water.

3. Peel the bananas and slice them thinly, about 1/8 inch thick.

4. Lightly dip each banana slice in the lemon juice mixture to prevent browning.

5. Lightly spray the air fryer basket with non-stick spray.

6. Place the banana slices in the air fryer basket in a single layer, making sure they do not overlap. You may need to cook them in batches to avoid overcrowding.

7. Air fry at 300°F (150°C) for 15-20 minutes, flipping the slices halfway through the cooking time. Keep a close eye on them to prevent burning.

8. Once the banana chips are golden brown and crispy, carefully remove them from the air fryer and place them on a wire rack to cool. They will continue to crisp up as they cool.

9. While the banana chips are cooling, prepare the smoothie by combining the frozen berries, banana, Greek yogurt, almond milk, and honey or maple syrup (if using) in a blender.

10. Blend until smooth and creamy.

11. Pour the smoothie into glasses.

12. Serve the banana chips alongside the smoothie as a delicious and nutritious breakfast.

Nutritional Information (per serving, based on 2 servings):

- **Calories: 250**
- **Protein: 6g**
- **Carbohydrates: 54g**
- **Dietary Fiber: 6g**
- **Sugars: 32g**
- **Total Fat: 3g**
- **Saturated Fat: 1g**
- **Sodium: 60mg**
- **Potassium: 600mg**

Lunch: Air Fryer Falafel with Tabouli

Ingredients:

For the Falafel:

- 1 can (15 oz) chickpeas, rinsed and drained
- 1/4 cup chopped fresh parsley
- 1/4 cup chopped fresh cilantro
- 1 small onion, finely chopped
- 2 cloves garlic, minced
- 1 teaspoon ground cumin
- 1 teaspoon ground coriander
- 1/2 teaspoon ground black pepper

- 1/2 teaspoon salt (optional, check with your dietitian)
- 1/4 teaspoon baking soda
- 1 tablespoon whole wheat flour
- 1 tablespoon olive oil
- Olive oil spray

For the Tabouli:

- 1/2 cup bulgur wheat
- 1 cup boiling water
- 1 cup finely chopped fresh parsley
- 1/2 cup finely chopped fresh mint
- 1/2 cup finely chopped tomato
- 1/4 cup finely chopped cucumber
- 1/4 cup finely chopped red onion
- 1/4 cup fresh lemon juice
- 2 tablespoons olive oil
- 1/4 teaspoon ground black pepper
- 1/4 teaspoon salt (optional, check with your dietitian)

Instructions:

Prepare the Falafel:

1. Put the chickpeas, black pepper, cumin, coriander, onion, garlic, parsley, cilantro, and salt (if

using) in a food processor. Pulse the mixture until it's thoroughly blended and coarse.

2. Pour the liquid into a basin and whisk in the whole wheat flour and baking soda. Blend the items thoroughly until they are properly blended.

3. Create little, 1.5-inch-diameter balls out of the mixture, then gently press them down to resemble patties.

4. Set your air fryer's temperature for three to five minutes at 375°F (190°C).

5. To keep the air fryer basket from sticking, lightly mist it with olive oil spray.

6. To ensure equal cooking, arrange the falafel patties in the air fryer basket in a single layer, allowing space between them. Apply a little layer of olive oil spray to the tops.

7. Cook the falafel for 12 to 15 minutes, turning them halfway through, or until they are crispy and golden brown.

8. Using tongs or a spatula, carefully take the falafel out of the air fryer and place it aside.

Prepare the Tabouli:

1. Transfer the bulgur wheat to a big bowl and cover it with the boiling water. Once the bulgur is soft and has absorbed the water, cover and let it sit for 15 to 20 minutes.

2. Use a fork to fluff the bulgur and let it cool slightly.

3. Top the bulgur with the chopped red onion, tomato, cucumber, mint, and parsley. Blend well.

4. Combine the lemon juice, olive oil, salt (if using), and black pepper in a small bowl. After pouring the dressing over the tabouli, toss to ensure uniform coating.

Assemble and Serve:

1. Present the tabouli and falafel patties side by side. If preferred, garnish with extra fresh herbs and slices of lemon.

Nutritional Information (per serving, based on 4 servings):

Falafel:

- **Calories: 180**
- **Protein: 6g**
- **Carbohydrates: 22g**
- **Dietary Fiber: 5g**
- **Sugars: 2g**
- **Fat: 7g**
- **Sodium: 200mg (varies with salt content)**
- **Potassium: 250mg**
- **Phosphorus: 100mg**

Tabouli:

- **Calories: 120**
- **Protein: 2g**
- **Carbohydrates: 18g**
- **Dietary Fiber: 4g**
- **Sugars: 2g**
- **Fat: 5g**
- **Sodium: 100mg (varies with salt content)**
- **Potassium: 300mg**
- **Phosphorus: 40mg**

Dinner: Air Fryer Zucchini and Black Bean Enchiladas

Ingredients:

- 2 medium zucchinis, diced
- 1 can (15 oz) black beans, drained and rinsed
- 1/2 cup corn kernels (fresh, canned, or frozen)
- 1 small onion, diced
- 1 clove garlic, minced
- 1 cup enchilada sauce (store-bought or homemade)
- 1 cup shredded low-fat cheese (optional)
- 8 small whole grain tortillas

- 1 tbsp olive oil
- 1 tsp ground cumin
- 1 tsp chili powder
- 1/2 tsp paprika
- 1/4 tsp black pepper
- 1/4 tsp salt
- Fresh cilantro for garnish (optional)
- Non-stick spray

Instructions:

1. For three minutes, preheat the air fryer to 375°F (190°C).
2. Heat the olive oil in a big skillet over medium heat. Add the chopped onion and simmer for 3–4 minutes, or until it turns transparent.
3. Add the minced garlic and stir until fragrant, about 1 more minute.
4. Fill the pan with the diced zucchini, black beans, and corn kernels. Mix everything together.
5. Add salt, black pepper, paprika, chili powder, and powdered cumin to the mixture. Sauté the zucchini for 5 to 7 minutes, or until they are soft.
6. Use a little amount of nonstick spray to coat a baking dish that fits within the air fryer basket.
7. To keep the baking dish from sticking, lightly coat the bottom with enchilada sauce.

8. Arrange the tortillas in a level fashion. Place a little amount of the black bean and zucchini mixture onto each tortilla, then firmly roll each one.

9. Slide the rolled tortillas into the baking dish, seam side down.

10. Evenly distribute the leftover enchilada sauce on top of the rolled tortillas.

11. Top the enchiladas with the low-fat cheese, if using, that has been shredded.

12. Insert the baking dish into the basket of the air fryer.

13. Air fry the enchiladas for 10 to 15 minutes, or until they are well cooked and the cheese is bubbling and melted, at 375°F (190°C).

14. Before serving, carefully take the baking dish out of the air fryer and allow the enchiladas to cool for a few minutes.

15. If preferred, garnish with fresh cilantro.

16. Serve warm and enjoy.

Nutritional Information (per serving, based on 4 servings):

- **Calories: 350**
- **Protein: 14g**
- **Carbohydrates: 45g**
- **Dietary Fiber: 10g**
- **Sugars: 5g**
- **Total Fat: 12g**

- **Saturated Fat: 3g**
- **Sodium: 600mg**
- **Potassium: 700mg**

CONCLUSION

Starting a kidney transplant journey necessitates several changes, the most important of which is adopting a diet that promotes the health of your new kidney and your general health. The Kidney Transplant Air Fryer Diet Cookbook attempts to make the transition easier and more pleasurable by offering tasty, healthy, and kidney-friendly dishes that can be prepared in an air fryer.

Throughout this cookbook, we've looked at several dishes that are tailored to your unique nutritional needs, with an emphasis on healthy grains, lean meats, and fresh fruits and vegetables. These recipes are intended not just to suit the nutritional needs of kidney transplant patients, but also to make your meals more enjoyable and satisfying. From crunchy air-fried veggies to sweet and savory nibbles, substantial main courses, and scrumptious desserts, there's something for everyone's tastes.

The air fryer has proven to be an important culinary appliance, with several health advantages.

It aids in the reduction of fat consumption, which is critical for heart health and weight management. Rapid cooking periods and high temperatures protect the nutrients in your food, ensuring that you get the most health advantages from each meal.

Furthermore, the air fryer's simplicity and ease of use promote regular good eating habits. Its adaptability enables you to experiment with a variety of dishes, minimizing dietary tiredness and making meals more fascinating and pleasurable.

Adopting a kidney-friendly diet entails not just making temporary modifications, but also embracing a new lifestyle that benefits your long-term health. This cookbook has given you the skills and knowledge you need to make healthy food choices for your kidneys and overall health. By incorporating these dishes into your everyday routine, you are actively working toward a better, happier life.

Key Takeaways

1. Balanced Nutrition: Eat a diet high in lean proteins, whole grains, fresh fruits, and vegetables, but limit sodium, potassium, and phosphorus consumption.

2. Healthy Cooking Methods: Use an air fryer to minimize fat consumption while maintaining the nutritional content of your meal.

3. Variety and Enjoyment: Experiment with new recipes and flavors to make your meals more interesting and pleasurable.

4. Ease and Consistency: Take use of the air fryer's ease to maintain constant healthy eating habits.

As you continue your kidney transplant journey, keep in mind that your diet is a vital instrument for guaranteeing the transplant's success and increasing your overall quality of life. The dishes in this cookbook are only the beginning. Continue to experiment with different foods while keeping your nutritional needs in mind.

Stay in touch with your healthcare team, especially your nutritionist, to adapt your diet to your unique needs and make modifications as needed. Regular check-ups and open contact with your healthcare providers can help you remain on track and handle any issues that may emerge.

I hope the Kidney Transplant Air Fryer Nutrition Cookbook has motivated you to confidently and enthusiastically manage your nutrition and health. By adding these dishes to your daily routine, you are not only fueling your body but also adopting a lifestyle that promotes long-term health and well-being.

Thank you for making this cookbook a part of your journey. May your meals be tasty, your health be robust, and your life be full of happiness and vigor.

Happy Good Health!

Made in United States
Orlando, FL
21 June 2025